PARENTING TRANSGENDER CHILDREN

PUBLISHED BY

STRONG FAMILY ALLIANCE

Second Edition

Copyright © 2022

Strong Family Alliance

All Rights Reserved.

All rights reserved. No part of this book may be reproduced in whole or in part without written permission from the author, except by a reviewer who may quote brief passages in a review; nor may any part be reproduced, stored in a retrieval system, transmitted in any form or by any means electronic, mechanical, including photocopying, recording, or other, without permission in writing from the author, except as provided by USA copyright law.

For more information, visit www.strongfamilyalliance.org

About Strong Family Alliance
Strong Family Alliance is a nonprofit organization with a simple mission—to save lives and preserve families by supporting parents of children coming out. Our website gives parents accurate information, insights on this challenging time for them and their child, ways to keep their child safe and healthy, and encouragement to lead with love and solve problems over time.

This book owes a huge debt
to the professional insights and guidance of my co-authors,
Shailagh Clarke, Ph.D., and Jennifer Gamewell, LPC.
Both serve as board members for Strong Family Alliance. Their
insights on everything from essential content to wording make this
book a valuable guide for parents and families.

We dedicate this book to all the families
who decide to love,
whatever the struggle.

TABLE OF CONTENTS

Chapter 1—Research About Transgender People....9
- Facts Help Dispel Myths

Chapter 2—Changes and Concerns 13
- Risks for Your Child
- The Stages of Coming Out
- Parent Actions That Help
- Parent Actions That Hurt
- Terms to Understand
- On Love and Freedom

Chapter 3—Finding Your Balance ....…...37
- The Journey for Parents
- Managing Emotions
- Tips for Supporting Your Child
- A Parents Story: Advice to Parents and Friends of Transgender Individuals

Chapter 4—Challenges Ahead ....…..57
- Understanding Transitioning
- Telling Others
- Relationships and Dating
- Myths That Stigmatize Transgender People
- Meeting Your Child's Significant Other

Chapter 5—Coming Out as the Parent…..........83
- Speaking Up: Independent Actions
- Telling Others: Coordinate with Your Child
- Working with a Counselor: Sharing in Private

Chapter 6—Moving Forward……………...……..99
- Tough Questions
- Issues of Faith
- Valuable Resources
- How to Have a More Meaningful Holiday

Prologue

Your child told you "I'm transgender," and you may be shaken and worried.

WE'RE HERE TO HELP.

If you're the parent of a child who recently disclosed that they are transgender (i.e. transgender, nonbinary, or in some way exploring their gender identity), you may be struggling, wondering how to respond, and worrying about the future. This guide will give you support, encouragement, information and resources that can help.

Our Mission

Strong Family Alliance is a nonprofit organization with a simple mission—to save lives and preserve families by supporting parents of children coming out. We give parents accurate information, insights on this challenging time for them and their child, ways to keep their child safe and healthy, and encouragement to lead with love and solve problems over time.

Our Goals

- Address the basic fears and conflicts for parents when a child comes out
- Provide up-to-date information about sexual orientation and gender identity
- Offer guidance on how to "do no harm" and keep their child safe
- Present answers to common initial questions and fears
- Use research-based information to provide needed support and clear steps for action
- Link to other positive resources for ongoing support

Chapter 1
Research About Transgender People

Facts Help Dispel Myths

There is a great deal of misinformation—even defamation—surrounding transgender people. Increasingly, research among trans individuals provides a more accurate picture of this community. Having good information is essential and helpful for parents.

Research focused on the trans community can provide insights, can dispel misconceptions, and can counterbalance some of the prejudices families encounter. From building their understanding of what transgender means to dispelling myths, accurate information is a bulwark for families and allies.

In late 2022, the Kaiser Family Foundation (KFF) and Washington Post produced The Washington Post/KFF Trans Survey in America[i]. Some of the key findings from that survey can be very helpful to parents.

Highlights of this survey follow, but please find the complete information on this survey online using the search term: KFF Washington Post Trans Survey.

Key Research Findings

1) Most trans adults view themselves as nonbinary or gender non-conforming.

How people identified was reported in the survey[ii]:

- 40% "trans nonbinary"
- 22% "trans, gender non-conforming"
- 22% "trans woman"
- 12% "trans man"
- 3% "some other way"

2) Most trans respondents did NOT have transition related medical treatments. Instead, transitioning can mean a variety of things[iii]:

- 77% changed their type of clothing
- 76% changed hairstyle or grooming to fit their identity
- 57% use a name different from their birth certificate
- 31% have used hormone replacement therapy (HRT) or puberty blocking hormones
- 16% have undergone gender-affirming surgery or surgically altered their appearance

3) While a trans person's identity may come as news to friends and family, most trans people knew they were trans early.[ii]

- 66% say they were younger than 18 when they knew their gender was different that their assigned sex
- 32% were aware when they were 10 or younger

4) Trans individuals tell others at many different ages, sometimes before they even have a word for it. [ii]

9%	10 years or younger
21%	11-17 years
32%	18-25 years
19%	26-40 years
5%	41-55 years
2%	56 and older
12%	Have not told anyone

5) Real hardship is faced by trans individuals in daily life.

It's important for families to know the hardship their trans loved one may face. Family support is crucial to a trans person's sense of safety and well-being. Families can listen, sympathize, and affirm their support for a trans loved one who reveals the pressures they face. Understanding these pressures are real, not imagined or exaggerated, is essential.

More findings from the survey reflect what these pressures are [ii]:

- 25% of trans adults have been physically attacked
- 64% have been verbally attacked
- 40% had unnecessary or invasive questions at work
- 21% were fired or denied a job or promotion
- 17% were refused service by a healthcare provider
- 13% were evicted or denied housing
- 21% of trans people of color were evicted or denied housing

There is much more information in this research report. You can find it online by searching 'KFF Washington Post Trans Survey.'

Most importantly, constantly build your knowledge of the trans community, your child's personal identity, and how you and your family can find the best future together.

References

i **The Washington Post.** *Nov. 10-Dec. 1, 2022, Washington Post-KFF Trans in America survey,* https://www.washingtonpost.com/tablet/2023/03/23/nov-10-dec-1-2022-washington-post-kff-trans-survey/

ii **The Washington Post.** *Most trans adults say transitioning made them more satisfied with their lives,* https://www.washingtonpost.com/dc-md-va/2023/03/23/transgender-adults-transitioning-poll/

iii **The Washington Post.** *6 key takeaways from the Post-KFF survey of transgender Americans,* https://www.washingtonpost.com/dc-md-va/2023/03/23/takeaways-post-kff-survey/

Chapter 2
Changes and Concerns

Most parents aren't sure how to react when their child discloses a different gender identity—simply because this isn't a focus until it touches their lives. Even parents who have close LGBTQ+ acquaintances or family members may find it difficult when their own child is involved. This is a powerful change in the family picture.

There are also two sides to this story of change. A child coming out to family members is emotionally vulnerable. Those who receive the news are often upset and overwhelmed. There will probably be missteps on both sides as they navigate this new territory.

This parent guide focuses on important information parents need to know how to help choose the best path for their family.

The good news: Staying connected, building communication, and working through change as a family can result in deeper relationships and better health for your child. While the challenges can be hard, many parents find they develop deeper, more honest, and more genuine relationships with their children as they work together through the changes they face.

> *"How could I not have known? I've come to learn and accept it was because she didn't fully know or understand it, let alone have the language to speak it out loud."*
> —Father of a transgender daughter
>
> *"Know that for every shred of despair, fear, anxiety, sense of failure you feel, it pales in comparison to what your child may have been going through."*
> —Mother of a transgender son

Risks for Your Child

Although it may feel difficult to support your child as they explore their gender identity (sometimes called "coming in") and disclose to others (also known as "coming out"), there is a higher risk to your child's health and safety if you don't support them. LGBTQ+ children who are rejected or cut off from family are more likely to experience physical and mental health problems.[1] Here are some statistics from research with transgender youth and adults:

Suicide

- LGBTQ+ youth rejected by family are 8 times more likely to attempt suicide.[1]
- Most teen suicides are impulsive with little or no planning and 70% occur in the victims' homes.[2]
- Of those transgender youth reporting at least one suicide attempt:
    - 50.9% were transgender female to male
    - 29.9% were transgender from male to female
    - 27.9% were adolescents who described themselves as "questioning"[3]
- A survey of 6000 transgender adults revealed that 45% of 18 to 24-year-olds attempted suicide, compared to 4.6% of the overall U.S. population.[4]

Violence and Bullying

- Approximately 3 out of 4 transgender and gender non-conforming youth hear their family make negative remarks about LGBTQ+ people.[5] More than half of transgender or gender non-conforming youth say they have been mocked by their family for their identity.[5]
- 84% of transgender youth said they do not always feel safe in the classroom.[5]
- More than half of young transgender people can *never* use the school restroom that aligns with their gender identity.[5]
- Nearly half (46%) of respondents were verbally harassed in the past year for being transgender.[6]
- Nearly one in ten (9%) were physically attacked in the past year for being transgender.[6]
- In 2022, over 150 anti-transgender bills were submitted in state legislatures.[7]

Drug and Substance Abuse

- Four percent (4%) of transgender respondents used illicit drugs (not including marijuana and nonmedical use of prescription drugs) in the past month.[6]
- Overall, 29% of transgender respondents reported illicit drug use, marijuana consumption, and/or nonmedical prescription drug use in the past month, which is nearly three times the rate in the U.S. population (10%).[6]

Parent support and strong family attunement can protect transgender kids, adolescents, and young adults. Continue reading to learn more about what they are experiencing and how your reactions can help or hurt.

The Stages of Coming Out

You may have just learned that your child is transgender (including nonbinary, gender expansive, and gender questioning). However, your child has probably been on this journey for months or years, also known as the "coming in" process. You have probably heard the term "coming out," which means telling others about orientation or gender identity. For transgender youth, the idea of "coming in" points to how they are developing or becoming aware of their sense of gender within themselves.

Knowing the stages they've been through is a first step to understanding their journey.[8]

Stage 1 – *Self Discovery as Transgender*

Becoming aware of gender identity can take time. Some people don't become aware until puberty sets in. Self-discovery may include confusion, anxiety, denial of feelings, and worries about being accepted. This internal conflict often results in continuing to appear as the gender that others expect, either due to preference or because circumstances require it.

Sometimes individuals attempt to "overcome" or deny their gender identity, particularly if they fear being condemned. LGBTQ+ people in general are often "in the closet" at this stage, which refers to keeping their identity to themselves. However, many seek out information online or through reading or from friends. This stage may be deeply, privately maintained until near puberty, until the emotional struggle requires action, or until the individual is more independent. Some individuals only come in as transgender adults.

The process can be different for everyone. Sometimes there are early indications, although "playing with dolls" or "being a tomboy" are not necessarily signs that a child is transgender.

Allow them to explore and follow their pace. Time will bring clarity: sometimes children may go back and forth, and others will be "persistent, insistent, and consistent" about their gender identity.

Stage 2 – *Disclosure to Others*

Disclosure is an ongoing process. The first step in this stage is sharing one's authentic self with a close friend or family member. Often this is a peer or close friend, and parents are not always the first to know. Disclosure may extend to more people over time. Rejection may cause a return to Stage 1, in which gender identity is kept private. However, a positive response from others can lead to higher self-esteem, greater self-acceptance, and most importantly, continued communication and openness.

In particular, the way parents respond when children disclose a different gender identity or questions about gender may deeply shape both the child's perspective about themself as well as the relationship with their parent. You don't have to have all the answers, but it is important to listen, express a desire to understand, and show love and affection.

For transgender persons who choose to socially or medically transition, their appearance, expression, pronouns, name change, and gender identity become more visible, and their privacy will diminish. Parental and family support at this time is particularly important to provide a safe harbor from discrimination or negative reactions they may encounter.

Stage 3 – *Socialization with Other Transgender People*

As a transgender child begins to find and connect with others who also identify as transgender or LGBTQ+, feelings of isolation and estrangement may diminish. A positive sense of self is strengthened by validation, education, support, and acceptance by a community of others who have shared experiences. Positive role models who are transgender are particularly important during this stage.

Stage 4 – *Positive Self-Identification*

The hallmark of this stage is feeling good about oneself, seeking positive relationships, and experiencing a sense of peace and fulfillment. At this point, the person begins to feel healthy and positive within their gender identity and the way they present themselves to others. Living as the gender with which they identify feels honest and true.

Stage 5 – *Integration and Acceptance*

This stage involves an openness and non-defensiveness about gender identity. Integration of this aspect of a person's identity may manifest itself in different ways, which could be anything from openly sharing their gender and their transition story with others to simply living as their authentic self without explanation or backstory.

Affirming relationships, family, friends, and communities of faith greatly impact an individual's ability to be fully integrated and self-accepting. At this stage, some individuals may become mentors or advocates for transgender or LGBTQ+ issues. It can affirm their success in claiming their identity to help others find resources, encouragement, and a personal path.

Stage 6 – *A Lifelong Journey*

Coming out as transgender does not happen just once. It is a lifelong process of discovering, accepting, and living within one's gender identity. In our society, we usually assume that everyone is heterosexual and lives in their sex assigned at birth. Transgender people must continually decide under what circumstances and with whom they will discuss their gender identity. Often their issues of safety and acceptance are complex, and building a supportive community is an ongoing process. Family support and encouragement continue to be a strengthening resource throughout their experiences. (Adapted from The Stages of Coming Out, by Richard Niolon, Ph.D.)

Notes and Journaling

Parent Actions That Help

> *"Somebody, your father or mine, should have told us that not many people have ever died of love. But multitudes have perished, and are perishing every hour--and in the oddest places!--for the lack of it."*
> ~Author James Baldwin

Many parents do not realize what an important role their comments, attitudes, and actions play in reducing risks for their transgender child. They are struggling with their own emotions. The good news: You can steer your child in a positive direction. What you choose to do (or not do) with and for your child can make a big difference for them right now and in their future.

Will you always love me?

This is the key question for transgender youth, whether they ask it directly or not. This question is far more important than the words "I'm trans" or "I'm nonbinary." It is essential that you express affection when your child discloses their gender to you, and that you continue to do so. Show your child that they are loved, even if you are struggling to accept this change in their identity. Warmth, respect, and displays of physical and emotional affection are more important now than ever. Don't ever hesitate to say, "I love you."

Keep Talking – and Listening

Your child may think that your silence on this topic means that you are angry with them. Parents who talk with and listen to their child or teen in a way that invites an open discussion about gender can help them feel loved and supported. It's important to let them talk and for you to sometimes raise the topic. This gives them permission to do so as well. Discuss news items, characters on TV or films, or a friend you know to open up discussion.

Even if it feels uncomfortable, keep up a flow of communication so your child feels comfortable continuing to talk to you. This includes talking with your child about their gender identity and experiences even when you are uncomfortable. Listening is as important as what you say. Ask how you can help and what your child needs. You don't need to have all the answers, you just need to be there for them.

> *"If they have a supportive family from the beginning, children who are transgender and gender-expansive don't experience higher rates of anxiety, depression, suicidal ideation or suicide compared with cisgender peers. Without family support, all those mental-health risks increase substantially. And having family use a child's preferred name and pronoun has been shown to be protective."*
>
> ~Tandy Aye, M.D., Stanford Medicine
>
> Associate Professor of Pediatrics

Make Sure Your Child Feels Affirmed and Supported

When your child discusses their gender identity, you may be tempted to try to figure things out by asking questions or suggesting alternative ideas and explanations. Instead, as one therapist for families with transgender kids says, "When your kid says they are transgender, just go with it." What does this look like? When your child brings up gender, refrain from arguing when they tell you who they are or what they need. More importantly, try to use the name or pronouns they prefer.

Although this might be the most difficult, using the name and pronouns your child requests may also be the most important choice parents can make to show transgender kids they are loved, accepted, and supported. Some other examples of actions that demonstrate your support and affirmation:[9]

- Listen in a way that invites open discussion about their gender. Be curious but not prying.
- Continue to include them in family activities.
- Help your child find support organizations and attend with them if appropriate.
- Take time to come to terms with your own feelings and reactions, so you can respond calmly and use respectful language.
- Try to get to know their friends and/or romantic partners.

Relationship is Paramount

When a child is transgender, parents have a cascade of emotions to deal with, but that takes time. Try to hold emotions in check, focus on your relationship, express love and affection, and let them know you are trying to understand. It's important to know your actions and words can support your child even as you struggle. Your child's perception of your acceptance or rejection has a huge impact.

Although it is vital for parents to sort through feelings and learn about what it means to be transgender, your child should not be the source of reassurance or information. As best you can, accept what your child tells you without asking why, when, what, and how, as these questions can feel like an interrogation. To the best of your ability, offer responses that do not include demanding explanations, asking for reasons, voicing doubts, or expressing sadness, worry, or fear.

The good news? Kids can tell if parents are trying, even when parents struggle or make mistakes. *According to recent research with transgender teens, the adolescents always rated their parents to be more supportive than the parents rated themselves.* "There are no medical side effects to listening and giving hugs or trying to use your child's preferred name and pronoun."[16] You will be adjusting to changes for a long time, but gestures of love, support, openness, and reassurance are supportive to your child. Your effort to build and sustain the relationship is key.

Stand Up for Your Child

You may hear negative comments made about your child or transgender people. How you speak *about* your child or transgender people can be as important as what you say directly *to* your child.

- Speak up with a different point of view and be aware your child is probably listening. Your words are a powerful witness to your support. Even if you are unsure, skeptical, or upset, a simple statement such as, "I don't think that's true" or "I don't know about that" when responding to negative comments or stereotypes will let your child know that you are on their side.
- Make it known that you will not accept discrimination, teasing, or insults to your child (e.g. "I don't think that's OK to say").
- Defend your child and advocate for them, even amid your own process of coming to acceptance about this (e.g. "They're figuring it out, I'm supporting them, and I hope you will too.").
- Insist that family members treat your child with respect, (e.g. "I know you don't understand, but please don't criticize/tease/deny/etc…").

Help Your Child Envision and Believe They Can Be a Happy Adult

Your acceptance and optimism helps your child envision a positive future and counteracts the hopelessness and sense of isolation that contribute to suicide and destructive behaviors. In one study, within families that were rated as very accepting, 92% of LGBTQ+ youth believed they would have good lives (92%) and most wanted to become a parent (69%).[10] While this statistic is not specific to families with transgender children, it does reflect the impact family acceptance can have on building optimism and a hopeful future outlook for youth who don't fit most cultural norms. Helping your child build a positive view of their future can be a strong support.

Doing this is not difficult. As with any child, it is important to encourage your child by helping them build on natural strengths, foster hope and optimism, avoid risky behaviors, and practice self-care both physically and emotionally.[11] Help them find activities, sports, clubs, or service work that can provide balance and variety as they learn skills. Ask about their dreams, what they would like to be, what their hopes are for education, work, and their adulthood or future. Building a mental picture of a positive future can help counterbalance current struggles.

Additional resources:

- "15 Reasons to Tell Your Child 'I Love You'" by Joshua Becker. *Becoming Minimalist.* (becomingminimalist.com)

- "How Parents Can Support Their Transgender Teens" by Erin Digitale. *Greater Good Magazine.* March 25, 2021.

- A list of more "Behaviors That Help" is located in Dr. Caitlin Ryan's booklet, Supportive families, healthy children: Helping families with lesbian, gay, bisexual & transgender children

Parent Actions That Hurt

Hearing your child question their gender can be an emotional shock, and both you and your child are vulnerable to strong emotions.

Parent comments, attitudes, and actions play a large role in how things turn out for their child.[1] Parent behaviors such as shaming or shunning are negative in any context. Many parents don't realize that even protective efforts can be felt as rejection by their child. Subtle actions, attitudes, words, or choices that communicate rejection to your child have been shown to be linked to both health and mental health problems:[1]

Abusive behaviors can include a variety of behavior that harms another person:[11]
- Aggression can include verbally belittling, dominating or insulting someone, criticism, arguing, controlling, or aligning against a family member.
- Lack of affection, such as the absence of verbal expressions of love, physical affection, encouragement, or time spent together.
- Neglect can include ignoring or not paying attention to someone, so that a person is not comfortable around some family members.
- Violence is considered physical harm and sexual abuse.[11]

It goes without saying that these actions are harmful. However, when they are aimed at your child's identity, they can be even more damaging. No matter what your reactions are, do not take them out on your child. What you choose to do (or not do) with and for your child can make a big difference.

Important Actions to Avoid

> *Family behaviors that try to change, prevent, deny or minimize their child's LGBTQ+ identity have a negative impact on their child's health and well-being and contribute to depression, suicide, illegal drug use and other serious health risks.*
> *~Family Acceptance Project,*
> *lgbtqfamilyacceptance.org*

Rejecting Your Child's Word That They are Transgender

"It's just a phase."

Disbelief or denying your child's identity is highly negative. Youth do not casually claim to be different than their sex assigned at birth, as it can bring challenges and even stigma. You may need time to adjust to it, but don't deny or minimize your child's disclosure. They trusted and loved you enough to be honest.

Refusing to Use Your Child's Chosen Name or Pronouns

"I know your name, I named you!"

Parents may feel strongly about their child's name, which is usually carefully chosen and may indicate family ties or tradition. But their own chosen name is an important marker for your child regarding how they identify. Their birth or given name is sometimes referred to as their "dead" name because it is not how they see themselves in their new identity. Using your child's chosen name is an important demonstration of support and acknowledgement and using their dead name can actually feel like a form of attack.

Changing their pronouns (he/she/they) can also be very difficult because habits are hard to break. However, your effort to try, even if you make mistakes, affirms to your child that you want to understand and support them in their new identity.

Hitting or Physically Hurting Your Child

"You deserved that!"

"The parental use of physical force is always risky…Damage to the parent/child relationship can be done if basic trust in safety with the parent is lost." [12]

Hurting with Words

"You're disgusting!"

Insulting is classified under emotional abuse. By definition, emotional abuse refers to any act by an adult that results in injuring a child's emotional health. When you yell at your child or throw insults at them, you are chipping away bits from their self-esteem. Insults come in many forms. Some of them include:

- Name-calling: "Are you stupid?"
- Shame: "You embarrass me…you are such a disappointment."
- Comparisons: "I wish you were more like your sister."
- Teasing in public: "Oh, he sucks at math; he's bottom of his class."
- Rejection: "Shut up and get out of my face."
- Extreme or negative criticisms: "You are a worthless embarrassment. Why can't you make me proud in even one thing?"[13]

> *"You may not be the only voice in your child's ear but make sure you're the best voice in your child's ear."*
>
> ~Dr. Phil

Excluding Your Child from Family Activities

"Not this time…"
"Your Aunt Maria won't understand, so maybe it's best if you stay home…"

Ostracizing someone does not just reduce feelings of belonging, it can also lower self-esteem, a sense of control, and a "sense of having a meaningful existence." [14] Ignoring, ostracizing, or marginalizing your child may inflict serious emotional pain and increase the risk of self-harming behaviors and despair. If you are concerned that a family member or friend may create discomfort for your child, a better tactic would be to discuss how the family will handle the situation. The plan should support, protect, and/or empower your child, and above all should feel comfortable for your child.

Blaming Your Child When Discrimination or Bullying Occur

"If you weren't trans, they wouldn't have…"
"If you worked a little harder to blend in…"

This is an example of a desire to protect coming across as rejection. Even if you believe it to be true, do not point to your child's gender identity as a reason that bad things happen to them, such as teasing, harassment, or loss of friendships.[1]

If your child is being bullied, ***they are the victim***. Taking the perspective of "you are bringing this on yourself" will only add shame to an already difficult experience. Empathizing and taking your child's side is an important show of support. Often all that is needed is to acknowledge how your child is feeling, rather than attempting to offer fixes, solutions, or changes your child should make.

Using Religion Against Them

"It's a sin."

It is deeply wounding to tell your child that he or she will be a disappointment to God or your religious community, particularly if your family is connected to a faith community. This will likely create self-hate or self-doubt within your child, but it will not create positive change. Please see the list of faith-based organizations on the Strong Family Alliance website to locate groups from many faiths and denominations that provide supportive information.

Notes and Journaling

Terms to Understand

Often parents don't absorb gender diversity terminology until the topic touches them personally. A first step in understanding and supporting your child is to gain a clear understanding of some common terms related to gender, including definitions and how they relate (or don't relate) to your child. Here's a basic list.

(The following is largely excerpted, with edits, from the GLAAD Media Reference Guide. Many additional terms are defined and described there.)

Cisgender - a person whose gender identity matches the sex they were assigned at birth. This male/female category applies to a large portion of society.

Gender Dysphoria - distress a person feels due to a mismatch between their gender identity—their personal sense of their own gender—and their sex assigned at birth. This is not always part of the transgender experience, but puberty may bring this feeling of mismatch to the surface.

Gender Expansive - Describes someone whose gender identity and/or gender expression expands beyond, actively resists, and/or does not conform to the current cultural or social expectations of gender, particularly in relation to male or female (see also nonbinary).

Gender Expression - How a person publicly expresses or presents their gender. This can include behavior and outward appearance such as dress, hair, make-up, body language, and voice. A person's chosen name and pronoun are also common ways of expressing gender. Others perceive a person's gender through these attributes.[15]

Gender Fluid - Describes someone whose gender identity is not fixed. Gender-fluid individuals prefer to remain flexible about their gender(s). Some dress in ways that reflect both genders at the same time, while others may express one gender one day and another gender another day.

Gender Identity - This is how someone sees themself. This is an individual's innate understanding of their own gender.

- NOTE: The terms *sexual orientation* and *gender identity* are often misused, but they are not the same and not interchangeable. A person of any gender identity could be sexually attracted to any type of person.

Gender Questioning - tentative gender identity label for a person who is in the process of figuring out how to describe and label their gender identity but has reason to think that they might be transgender or nonbinary.

Nonbinary - an adjective used by people who experience their gender identity and/or gender expression as falling outside the two (i.e. binary) categories of man and woman. Many nonbinary people also call themselves transgender and consider themselves part of the transgender community. Others do not.

Queer - An adjective used by some people, particularly younger people, whose sexual orientation is not exclusively heterosexual. Typically, for those who identify as queer, the terms lesbian, gay, and bisexual are perceived to be too limiting and/or requiring them to label themselves. Once considered a pejorative term, queer has been reclaimed by some LGBTQ+ people to describe themselves. However, it is not a universally accepted term even within the LGBTQ+ community.

Sexual orientation - This is about who a person is attracted to. This is a person's enduring physical, romantic, and/or emotional attraction to another person.

Trans - Shorthand for transgender.

Transgender - An umbrella term that describes people whose gender identity differs from the sex they were assigned at birth. Being transgender is *not dependent upon physical appearance or medical procedures*. It's an identity. A person can call themself transgender the moment they realize that their gender identity is different from the sex they were assigned at birth. People who are transgender may also use other terms, in addition to transgender, to describe their gender more specifically.

Transition - The process a person undertakes to bring their gender expression and/or their body into alignment with their gender identity. It is a complex process that occurs over a long period of time and the exact steps involved in transition will vary from person to person. Chapter 3 provides more detail about the variety of transition steps.

Some transgender people may not feel they need to take any transition steps at all, while others may wish to transition but cannot due to cost, underlying medical conditions, and/or fear of consequences from transphobic family, employers, etc. A person can call themselves transgender the moment they realize that their gender identity is different from the sex they were assigned at birth, whether they take transition steps or not.

- **Social transition** - Telling family, friends, and co-workers, using a different name, using different pronouns, dressing differently, starting or stopping wearing make-up and jewelry, etc.
- **Legal transition** - Changing your name and/or sex marker on documents like a driver's license, passport, Social Security record, bank accounts, etc.
- **Medical transition** - Hormone therapy and/or one or more surgical procedures.

(NOTE: Occasionally additional terms and definitions arise, such as pansexual, omnisexual, two spirit, and more. This can lead to complicated indicators such as LGBTQIA2S+. For simplicity, we have focused on terms most applicable to transgender issues. However, evolving definitions can be found on the websites of CDC.gov, the Mayo Clinic, and even online dictionaries.)

**On Love and Freedom
by Janet Gattis Duke
(From Strong Family Alliance Blog)**

Amid the pandemic, I saw an uptick in new visitors to our Strong Family Alliance website – something more usual during holidays when families gather. Research shows it takes most families about two years to find a new balance as a child comes out. This made me think about things that were valuable to my LGBTQ+ daughter and our relationship in the years since she came out.

Determination to love was the most important. That sounds negative. But I found love was often an act of will. When I was confused or hurting, it was be hard to be loving. When I was worried or fearful, I meant to love but I could come across as angry.

Being a parent is hard work and sometimes it is guesswork. But there were added challenges when parenting an LGBTQ+ teen. I encountered situations with a twist and had to work through them. For instance, dating is a normal part of growing up, but with an LGBTQ+ child it was more complicated. Do the other parents know? Is it safe where they are going?

Sleepovers that would have been no problem became a challenge. Schools for all grades were a consideration, from teacher support to extra-curricular choices. Selecting a college suddenly included more than academics or affordability. (If you are in this process, please see our section on Colleges, Scholarships and Educational Resources for LGBTQ+ on www.strongfamilyalliance.org)

I found determination to love could change my attitude. I rejected the self-pity of "why is this so hard" or "if only things were *normal*" and intentionally choose a different point of view: "we are in this together and I am on your side." That made all the difference.

It took time to process the loss of my predictable future —a process most parents face. I had many dreams for the future that had to be reimagined. I often slipped back into the worry cycle and had to intentionally refocus. That is where determination came in.

Along the way I learned about the importance of freedom. Not for me but for my child. I often gave guidance that had worked for me. Ideas about clothing, making friends, dealing with hurts, etc. I was guilty of over-advising. It is one thing to talk over options, it is another to constantly say "you should…"

Things that worked for my time and situation were different for her. I had to learn to give her freedom to choose. I had to learn to help only if asked. I found that not fully understanding the challenges she faced day to day made me a better parent. I had to listen more. I had to learn from her. I had to let her take the lead in her own choices and in the process we grew closer.

Other parents say their closeness increases as well. Working through their challenges together brings their family closer. They become more honest with each other. They develop better communication. They learn to find new options and solutions that work for them. They find supportive communities, churches, and schools. They build a stronger, more connected and understanding family.

Two things I learned worked for us: determination to love and granting my child freedom to lead her own life. My hope is that each family finds the techniques that help them build their best future together. That during any other challenges, they stay well, grow closer and discover new possibilities.

REFERENCES

1. Ryan, C., Huebner, D., Diaz, R. M., & Sanchez, J. (2009). Family rejection as a predictor of negative health outcomes in White and Latino lesbian, gay, and bisexual young adults. *Pediatrics, 123,* 346-352.

2. SPEAK: Suicide Prevention Awareness Education for Kids. *Suicide facts.* http://www.speakforthem.org/facts.html

3. Toomey R. B., Syvertsen A. K., & Shramko M (2018). Transgender Adolescent Suicide Behavior. *Pediatrics*, 142(4):e20174218

4. Haas, A. P., Rodgers, P. L., & Herman, J. L. (2014). *Suicide attempts among transgender and gender non-conforming adults: Findings of the national transgender discrimination study.* American Foundation for Suicide Prevention, The Williams Institute. 10.13140/RG.2.1.4639.4641

5. Human Rights Foundation. *Dismantling a culture of violence: Understanding anti-transgender violence and ending the crisis, Updated 2021.* Human Rights Campaign. https://reports.hrc.org/dismantling-a-culture-of-violence

6. National Center for Transgender Equality. *2015 US Transgender Survey.* https://transequality.org/sites/default/files/docs/usts/USTS-Full-Report-Dec17.pdf

7. Freedom for All Americans. *Legislative Tracker: Anti-Transgender Legislation.* https://freedomforallamericans.org/legislative-tracker/anti-transgender-legislation/. Accessed on April 24, 2022.

8. Niolon, R. *The stages of coming out.* Gay/Lesbian Resources. http://www.psychpage.com/learning/library/gay/comeout.html

9. Ryan, C. (2009). *Supportive families, healthy children: Helping families with lesbian, gay, bisexual & transgender children.* San Francisco, CA: Marian Wright Edelman Institute, San Francisco State University.

10. Ginsburg, K.R. & Jablow, M.M. (2005). *Building resilience in children and teens, 2nd Ed.: Giving kids roots and wings.* American Academy of Pediatrics: Elk Grove Village, IL.

11. Hall, E. D., (March 27, 2017). *Why family hurt Is so painful: Four reasons why family hurt can be more painful than hurt from others.* Psychology Today. https://www.psychologytoday.com/us/blog/conscious-communication/201703/why-family-hurt-is-so-painful

12. Pickhardt, C. (September 29, 2014). *Parenting and the use of physical force: Better to talk out than physically act out to try to get the parental way.* Psychology Today. https://www.psychologytoday.com/us/blog/surviving-your-childs-adolescence/201409/parenting-and-the-use-physical-force

13. Being the Parent. *Insulting children – The worst parenting technique.* https://www.beingtheparent.com/insulting-children-the-worst-parenting-technique/

14. Williams, K. D., Nida, S. A. (2011). Ostracism: Consequences and coping. *Current Directions in Psychological Science, (20),* 71-75.

15. Ontario Human Rights Commission. (April 14, 2014). *Policy on preventing discrimination because of gender identity and gender expression.* https://www.ohrc.on.ca/en/policy-preventing-discrimination-because-gender-identity-and-gender-expression

16. Digitale, E. (March 8, 2021). *5 Questions: Tandy Aye on what transgender teens need from their parents.* Stanford Medicine News Center https://med.stanford.edu/news/all-news/2021/03/how-parents-can-help-their-transgender-teens.html

Chapter 3
Finding Your Balance

As a transgender child "comes in" to their new identity, parents often find themselves sorting through complex emotions. They may not know what to expect or how to deal with their feelings. Or, after they have adjusted, they may find their balance is upset again and again.

These are common experiences, and knowing what to expect and how to keep helping your child can be a relief. Hopefully, this chapter can help you find you balance.

Few organizations focus on the struggle parents face in navigating these changes in the family, but ours does. We hope you'll visit the Strong Family Alliance website often.

The Journey for Parents

> *"The greatest freedom for me came when I realized that (her) being transgender was not a defect but a gift in my life...I have grown closer to my daughter and seen her becoming happier every year. This journey has made me a better father and a better person."*
>
> *~Oregon father of a transgender daughter*

It can be a shock to learn a child is transgender, and there are definite stages that most parents experience. The stages below do not always happen in order—or just once—and some may not occur at all. Some stages pass quickly, others slowly. But the following stages can represent the struggle to accept an enormous change in your family.

Many life events can trigger feelings you thought you had worked through already. For instance, if your child begins to date, moves away to college, or encounters bullying or a hurtful comment, you may feel as if you have gone backwards to one of the earlier stages. This is common. Allow yourself to work through those feelings and regain your balance.

Stage 1 – Denial

Initial denial or disbelief is common. Although many of us might wonder if our child is transgender even before they tell us, usually we suppress and deny this possibility out of fear of what the truth might mean to our family, or our child's future.

Even after a transgender child comes out, parents may hope that this is a phase, a rebellion, or an experiment. However, when a child takes the major step of telling a parent they have a different gender identity, it is important to take them at their word.

This can be difficult, because it means truly facing what being transgender could mean for the child and for you. Most people don't focus on understanding what being transgender means until it touches them personally. You may find yourself in new and uncharted territory.

Stage 2 – Grief

Grief is sadness about a loss. We may grieve the loss of the child we "knew" and the future we imagined. We mourn the disappearance of the life we envisioned for them. It takes time to grieve the death of the dreams for our child that center around gender-specific life events. For example, a father may experience sadness related to his expectation that he would walk his daughter down the aisle at her wedding.

As with many changes, over time new dreams are built and new hopes arise. Some hopes may remain but broaden, such as changing the hope for a good wife/husband to hope for a good partner/spouse. But the fundamental hopes and dreams can endure, such as love and happiness, career success, or starting a family.

Stage 3 – Blame/Guilt

Many parents feel the need to determine a reason why, which may lead to guilt or blame. We blame ourselves, wondering if we did something "wrong." We blame our children for "changing" and for forcing us to readjust our vision. We might even blame their friends, partners, or other transgender people, incorrectly believing that our child was drawn to this identity through the influence of others.

Research shows being gay or transgender is not the result of any specific choice, behavior, or event. A shift from the sex assigned at birth is not an illness, disease, or choice. Gender identity is a variant of human sexuality and development that arises as the result of complex interactions of biological, genetic, and hormonal factors. In addition, there is a growing understanding, especially among younger people, that gender is more like one point along a spectrum. That male and female are just two of many possible ways gender can be expressed and lived.

Stage 4 – Fear

We fear what we do not understand and for most parents there are many unknowns when it comes to what it means to be transgender. We fear reactions from others and telling what may feel like a difficult truth. We fear being judged and losing our friends, family, and faith community. We fear the hatred, violence, and discrimination our transgender child may encounter and endure. All of these are realistic possibilities for both parent and child, which makes it even more important to support each other and navigate the changes together.

Sometimes, fear may be justified. If you sense a friend or family member will be hostile, you can choose to protect your child by remaining silent about their transgender identity. This is not necessarily a bad thing as long as it feels supportive to your child.

Your child should determine who knows and when to tell, for they will bear the result. A transgender child may feel safest with just friends and family knowing. Or they may pursue appearance changes that make a more public statement. Whatever their level of expression, it's important to let them set the pace and take the lead. Follow their cues. Ask if you are in doubt. For example, "Would you mind if I tell Aunt Kay you are transgender?"

If your child is open, it is important to keep pace and show support. When a family is not open about their child's identity it is sometimes referred to as being in the "Second Closet." This can be a good thing if the child needs privacy, but it can be a very bad thing if the child views it as the silence of shame.

Stage 5 – Anger

We may feel angry at…

- Society or governments for allowing or promoting discrimination.
- Ourselves for not recognizing the truth sooner.
- Our child for causing upheaval in our family.
- Other family members when feelings intensify either for or against the transgender child.
- God for "allowing" our precious loved ones to be transgender, because their lives may be more difficult.
- "Why me?" and "Why my child?" are common feelings.
- Our religious community for rejecting or condemning transgender people and their families.

It's important to deal with your own anger and not direct it toward your child. Don't expect your child to explain everything to you. Information can help combat anger, and educating yourself is a good first step, but this is your work to do. There are several books in our resources list that may be helpful to understand your experience. Talking with trusted family or friends or seeking counseling are also good options to help deal with anger.

It may help to recall that your child has honored you by trying to be truthful and honest. Deciding not to hide anymore and a longing to live more honestly and authentically are strong motivations for many transgender individuals. Try to honor them by managing your emotions as you grow your understanding.

Stage 6 – Self-Realization

With this stage comes the realization that it is we, not our child, who must change. How?
- Redraw our family picture to include this new reality
- Support our child and the family they have or will create
- Surround ourselves with other loving parents and friends
- Find a nurturing faith community
- Learn all we can and help others learn as well

Family members may not come to this understanding at the same pace, but as each person accepts and supports the transgender child, the child will gain an increased sense of safety and community.

Stage 7 – Acceptance

Quite simply, this means loving your transgender child, not in spite of who they are, but just as they are.

Your acceptance of your transgender child creates a safe space where they can build a good life and become their best self. They still need things parents can so powerfully provide, such as love, encouragement, understanding, and a hopeful view of the future. In addition, many parents find their child is happier, more resilient, and more open and connected with them as family acceptance grows.

You may become a resource for other families by helping them find support. It is also often helpful to read stories from parents and families who have shared your experience. You can read stories from other parents on our "Family Stories" page on the Strong Family Alliance website. When you are ready, consider sharing your story as well.

At the end of this guide, we include a reprinted article about raising a transgender son to provide the view from a parent further along in this journey.

Managing Emotions

Different Roles: Parent and Child

There are two parts to re-balancing family relationships with this powerful change in the family picture:

- **The Parent's Role**—finding your own path, keeping your balance, and helping all the children involved, which may include siblings.
- **The Child's Role**—learning how to live positively with the challenges of their newly shared identity.

However off-balance you may feel when your child comes out, it's important to avoid laying your fears and worries on your child. Healthy parenting suggestions include:

Avoid "Venting" to Your Child

It's essential that your child not become a lightning rod for the many emotions you may feel. Concerns about the future can be heightened now, and it's important not to use your child as a place to work through your emotions. This section has valuable insights into the parent experience and suggestions below offer alternative ways to handle your feelings.

Find Personal Support

- Join a support group such as PFLAG. Local chapters in many areas provide support for families and individuals. Many parents and families have been in your situation, and their experiences and insight can be a tremendous resource.

- Confide in someone you trust, such as a close friend or a supportive sibling, about what you're going through. Make sure this person is a positive and encouraging resource.
- Consider counseling. Sometimes the best resource is at arm's length. A therapist is outside the situation and can provide perspective. Contact your state or local mental health agency for help finding a counselor if you don't know where to start or check out online resources such as www.goodtherapy.org, www.betterhelp.com, or the Therapist Finder at psychologytoday.com. Be sure to ask about their experience with transgender issues.
- Write in a journal. Writing helps you express your feelings, organize your thoughts, and will become a record of your progress over time.
- Practice self-care. Exercise and good health habits are important for your whole family. Be a role model.

Get Informed

Learn all you can about your child's new identity and the challenges they may face. Don't expect your child to educate you. They may still be learning themselves. Focus on positive resources and up-to-date information. Our Resources page at www.strongfamilyalliance.org has pointers. The time you spend learning has many benefits:

- Knowledge reduces fear and worry.
- Information helps you navigate situations and make decisions with more confidence and compassion.

Listen, Listen, Listen

You need to know what your child is facing. If they can come to you first, they are safer. It may be difficult initially but keeping communication open—primarily through listening—strengthens your understanding and relationship.

Practice **WAIT** — **W**hy **A**m **I T**alking.

Consider using questions or phrases that encourage them to talk:
- Tell me more about that.
- How did that make you feel?
- What was that like?
- Can you tell me more?
- Summarize what they said to show you are listening.

Help the Family Keep its Balance

- Maintain the ordinary. Keep routines going for school, teams, or extracurricular activities.
- Find opportunities for family participation. Activities you can do with all or part of the family help maintain relationships and normalcy. This can be as simple as movies, athletic events, outings, or service projects.

Support Siblings

- Sibling reactions vary greatly. If they need support or education, help them find it.
- If your child is ready for siblings to know, don't forget to talk with your other children about this change and how they feel about it or how it affects them.
- Brothers or sisters are sometimes the first to know, but not always. If it's news to them, they may have many of the emotions you experience and will need to work through those.
- Siblings may be embarrassed, or fear others will think they are LGBTQ+ because their brother or sister is transgender.
- It's important they understand the risks their sibling faces and why family support is essential.
- Share our website with them if it's age appropriate—it's a good starting point if they are struggling.

Help Your Child Connect

Help your child find positive connections with other transgender and LGBTQ+ youth. Isolation leads to feelings of depression and shame. Possible resources include:

- School Clubs—many schools have GSA clubs (Gay Straight Alliance/Genders and Sexualities Alliance) that work with a sponsoring teacher and parents to plan events, service projects, and support meetings. If your school doesn't have a chapter, talk with a counselor about starting one.
- Online resources from groups such as PFLAG (Parents and Friends of Lesbians and Gays), GLSEN (focused on LGBTQ+ issues in K-12) and many others.
- Look for local drop-in or meetup programs. Some communities have church or organization-sponsored after school or social hour resources.
- Find a support group. Organizations such as PFLAG and transfamilies.org hold meetings for both parents and youth.

Work on the Environment in Your Family and Home

- Learn more about prejudice and discrimination based on such differences as race, sexual orientation, gender identity/expression, and religion.
- Monitor your own beliefs about LGBTQ+ people and how they influence your child.
- Be a positive role model for your child on respectful treatment of transgender and LGBTQ+ individuals in your community: teachers, coaches/athletes, neighbors, co-workers and public figures.
- Assume that LGBTQ+ people are in a group even if they have not identified themselves. This can include parties, meetings, teams, classrooms, or any gathering.

- Stand up for all LGBTQ+ people—If you hear a painful joke or derogatory comment, push back. If your child hears you, it's a powerful affirmation. If not, tell them about it anyway. It can mean a lot to know you stand up for them. Examples of verbal pushback include:

    o I don't think that's funny.
    o That comment could hurt someone.
    o I disagree.
    o That's a hateful thing to say.
    o My child is LGBTQ+.

Notes and Journaling

Tips for Supporting Your Child

> *As we began to share her truth, with her blessing, we learned what the important people in our lives think – and the majority of them reacted in love to the news. We discovered that we no longer cared so much about what the non-supportive people think."*
>
> ~Mother of a transgender daughter

Be open. Be supportive. Be informed.

Appreciate when a young person comes out to you.

Coming out is scary. Your transgender child has probably tested you with a series of trials over time—listening to your comments, watching how you respond to topics, jokes or slurs. Based on your previous responses, they decided you can be trusted. There may still be fear of rejection, ridicule, and abuse, but they are hoping the parent they love and depend on can be counted on again. When someone comes out to you, your primary task is to respect their courage and honesty, thank them for trusting you, and continue caring for them.

Respect confidentiality.

When someone shares their gender identity or sexual orientation with you, you have received a confidence which must be respected. Breaching this trust can be emotionally and physically damaging. Be guided by the wishes of the person who confided in you. Coming out it is a gradual process and the timing of who knows and when should be controlled by the person coming out.

Examine your own biases.

Male and female roles are strongly defined in our culture: boy or girl, pink or blue, transformers or dolls, players or cheerleaders, and many other messages constantly define male/female roles. Despite modern trends, most of us are products of a gender rigid society.

You can't be free of that just by deciding to be—it takes an intentional effort to break free of assumptions. Try to inform yourself—read, seek reliable, factual resources, and talk with your loved one about their experience and point of view. It's a gift you give yourself and your child.

Learn where to seek help.

Familiarize yourself with the supportive referral agencies and counselors in your denomination and area. LGBTQ+ helplines and support groups can connect you with experienced people and organizations.

Maintain a balanced perspective.

Sexuality and gender identity make up a small but truly important part of every person's identity. Your transgender child is still the same person you have known and loved for years. That person is still there and cares enough about you to be deeply honest about themselves.

They have trusted you with the most personal and risky information they can share, and they are hoping you will still love them. It's urgently important to do so. However big this difference may seem to you, the larger person, the child you love, is still there. Don't let a smaller part overshadow the whole.

Understand the meaning of sexual orientation and gender identity.

Sexual orientation and gender identity are not the same thing. Sexual orientation is about *attraction to another person*. This describes romantic, emotional, or sexual feelings toward others. People do not choose who they are attracted to, they simply are.

Gender identity is about *self-perception*. This is a person's inner sense of being male, female, somewhere in between, or neither. This is an awareness of who they are, rather than who they are attracted to, and is a separate issue with unique complexities.

Be supportive.

Help connect the young person to transgender resources, support groups, and alliances. Many lesbian, gay, bisexual, and transgender youth feel alone, afraid, and ashamed because of religious, societal, and familial pressures. You can assist by listening with care to their feelings and concerns, offering a supportive and nonjudgmental presence, and remembering they are valuable to the world.

Anticipate some confusion.

LGBTQ+ youth receive so many messages that their orientation or gender identity is strange or sinful, they may be confused or even attempt to deny who they are. While many youths are aware of their sexual orientation and gender identity even before early adolescence, this awareness can take years to fully integrate. Often, they are in the middle of adolescence when their self-image is rapidly changing.

You can help by:

- Affirming to them that their feelings are normal and natural.
- Allowing them to wonder about themselves and try on different ideas. This is typical of the teen years when most people struggle with questions of who we are and how we fit in the world. This is no different for transgender youth. Listening to their thoughts builds communication and can provide insight. Parents often find themselves jumping to "will my child want surgery?" when often gender identity changes begin (and sometimes end) with changing pronouns and name.
- Remembering that no one can be talked into or out of the gender they identify with, even if it is not the one assigned at birth.

> *"I did a lot of grieving over the loss of the image I had of my only son in my mind and heart. I had to deal with the loss of my previous perception of our relationship and the loss of my expectations of the future...Eventually I found friends, relatives and colleagues I felt safe to talk with about this change in our lives. I also chose to get some therapy to help myself process my feelings and to be the best parent I could be to our daughter."*
> *~Mother of a transgender daughter*

Help, but do not force.

If you are comfortable with your gender, you may not fully understand what it means to be different in ways transgender individuals experience. We often urge young people into behavior, clothing or experiences that are familiar to us or that served us well in the past. We also urge them toward things we would do or use because those are comfortable to us and well known.

The best clues for how to help will come from your loved one. Don't force them into your frame of reference to make it easier for you to understand. Remember, teen years are often a time for experiments in appearance, activities, and interests. Be open and patient.

Challenge anti-trans remarks.

Speak up whenever you hear anti-trans or anti-LGBTQ+ jokes or disparaging language and try to remember to *function as if there is a transgender youth in your midst* (even if you don't think there is). Your words and example will send the message that offensive remarks will not be tolerated, and that you are affirming of LGBTQ+ people and their families. You will also signal to LGBTQ+ youth that you are a safe person with whom to talk. Don't perpetuate injustice and ignorance by remaining silent. Defend others' dignity.

Source: Parents Reconciling Network. (2014) *Tips for relating to lesbian, gay, bisexual, transgender, questioning, queer & intersex youth.* Reconciling Ministries Network. https://rmnetwork.org/wp-content/uploads/2020/12/prn-supporting-youth.pdf (Revised by permission.)

Notes and Journaling

A Parents Story:
Advice to Parents and
Friends of Transgender Individuals

Our son is transgender. We welcomed him into the world twenty-six years ago as a daughter, but he is our son. What does that mean? Three years ago, he had surgery to give himself a more masculine body. Two years ago, he began hormone treatment, which led to male puberty. He changed his name to Jeremy and asked that we use male pronouns. We are proud of him and love him.

But we have a long way to go. It is still exceedingly difficult to be transgender in America today. As the parent of a transgender man, I am sometimes asked for advice. I offer the following as a way to help others who have someone trans in their lives.

1. Know that your transgender friend or family member is an individual, not just a representative of the transgender community. He or she or they is the same person as before transitioning. Whatever you talked about before will still be of interest afterwards. They may or may not be politically active in the LGBTQ+ community. They may be open about being transgender, or they may want to simply live their life as the gender that matches their identity. Take your lead from your friend or loved one.

2. Listen with an open mind and heart. You won't know how to best support your child or friend or sibling or parent if you don't listen and do so in a nonjudgmental manner. Someone transitioning is on a journey that requires tremendous courage. Respect that and believe that your friend or loved one is trying their best to guide you as to what they need from you. Know that this will get easier over time.

3. Use whatever name and pronoun is requested. A transgender individual will have spent a lot of time and emotional energy deciding on a new name and pronouns. Don't worry if the pronouns aren't familiar to you or if they don't sound grammatically correct. Don't worry if you make mistakes; my son only gets annoyed if he feels as if someone isn't trying.

4. Recognize that everyone's journey is different. Many articles have been written about children who have known from the time they were toddlers that they were a different gender from how they were identified at birth. Some people don't figure things out until much later, and their journeys don't follow a straight line. There is no one right way to be transgender.

5. Educate yourself. Watch videos. Read books. Explore articles on the Internet. More resources appear every day, and they can be a tremendous help. Ask your transgender friend or family member what websites they found to be most helpful and then visit those yourself. Likely you will find stories similar to your own.

6. Accept your own feelings. It is okay to feel a sense of loss. You may be angry. Or overwhelmed. You may ask, "Why is this happening?" Everyone reacts differently and on their own schedule. Keep in mind that recognizing your own feelings will help you better support your transgender loved one. But also keep in mind that a child may be hurt by hearing you work through those feelings. Remember to always show your child support.

7. Become a part of an LGBTQ/ally community. You are not alone. There are some wonderful groups of people who have been fighting for LGBTQ+ rights for a long time and are extraordinarily welcoming of friends and family of transgender individuals. Go online and look for organizations in your area. Not only will you find they help you through what could be a difficult journey, you will also find that you make some new friends.

8. Express support—strongly and frequently. Transgender children are among the most bullied in our schools. Trans teenagers often suffer from depression and anxiety. Over 40 percent have tried to die by suicide. Transgender adults are all too often the targets of hatred and violence. This is a difficult path. Nobody follows it lightly; they do so because it is who they are.

Expressing your love and support can go a long way toward making things easier. And, if your trans friend or loved one has gone public, speak up openly to show your acceptance. Every time we share our stories about the transgender people we care about, we build awareness. Hopefully, with that awareness will come greater acceptance.

9. Be joyful. The journey, although hard in some ways, will also be filled with joy. I will not pretend that there aren't difficult moments. But the joyous times are many. The realization that I'd had a son all along. The pride when I recognized the courage my son demonstrates every single day. The love that I feel for him. The incredible happiness that my son's transition has brought to him.

When he looked over this article for me, his response was, "I'm glad that you ended with 'Be joyful.' Transitioning is the most affirming thing a person can do. While scary, allowing yourself to be one hundred percent yourself is joyful indeed."

Jo Ivester is the author of the award-winning memoir, "The Outskirts of Hope." Initially published with Huffington Post, her article is reprinted here as modified in her book, *Once a Girl, Always a Boy*, published by She Writes Press.

Chapter 4
Challenges Ahead

> *Our daughter especially has opened my eyes to a lot of thinking about life in different terms and different ways and I think that's really positive, being able to learn from her. I wouldn't have it have it any other way. I'm just thrilled. I feel like it's a privilege and a pleasure that I would never have anticipated when we had our children."*
> ~Anonymous, mother of a lesbian daughter

Millions of parents have come to terms with this change in their family and many develop deeper, closer relationships with their children. Like many highly emotional transitions, a positive outcome is often determined by your attitude and actions. Start here to learn about some common challenges and how you can navigate this change in your family.

According to a 2013 Pew Research Center survey[1] of LGBTQ+ adults 18+, about 54% of "all or most of the important people in their life" know they are LGBT. Not all youth come out to their families. Consider that your transgender child coming out to you shows:

- a desire to be honest and open with you
- trust in you as a parent and safe confidante
- a wish to have a closer relationship
- a strong need to live in their chosen gender identity

You and your child may be out of step on this journey. Transgender youth have probably been considering their identity for years. You may be on a steep learning curve. We hope this section can provide some fundamental background and strategies to help keep your relationship with your transgender child strong.

Transitioning

Transitioning is the process a person undertakes to bring their gender expression and/or their body into alignment with their gender identity. Transitioning is a complex process that occurs over a long period of time, and the steps involved in transition will vary from person to person.

One of the most common misunderstandings about transgender individuals is that they are all the same. How they transition, the degree to which they transition, the timing and pace, and how they express their identity all vary tremendously. This article is not a list of all the options, but it can be helpful to understand transitioning as rough categories rather than one event or path.

"Coming In" or the personal transition

Most human cultures are heavily gendered. There are strong patterns and expectations of boys/girls and women/men. Transgender individuals live in this environment and know very well what patterns may be expected of them based on their birth gender.

The personal transition is a process that begins when individuals experience dissonance between the patterns surrounding them, how others view and react to them, and how they feel about themselves. This can occur at any time, from early childhood to puberty to adulthood.

Playing with trucks or dolls in early childhood is not an indicator. Most children experiment at young ages with a variety of toys or mimicking adults or characters on TV or in movies. What is more important is the duration and constancy of the role the person chooses.

For parents trying to understand their child, it's helpful to know how to evaluate the child's view. A key is time, and that the person is:

- *Persistent* – maintaining their identity over time
- *Insistent* – pushing back against efforts to change their view and adamant about their identity
- *Consistent* – the person is constant in their description or claiming of their identity

For adolescents this personal transition can take many forms. Sometimes it occurs around puberty but not always. It's a time of reflecting on how they see themselves compared to how they are perceived in the world around them.

When they become firm in their self-image and want to portray that in their daily life they may share with a friend or trusted family member that they are transgender. Peers or online acquaintances may know before family members. How and when transgender youth talk with family can vary from email or text to letters to voicemails to one-on-one conversations and more.

Social transition

Social transitioning refers to when the transgender person begins living their identity around others. Telling family, friends and co-workers is often a start. Individuals may begin using a different name, one they chose for themselves that is meaningful to them. Pronouns may change and they ask for others to use the chosen pronouns. They may begin to dress differently, groom differently, add/stop/change their jewelry, makeup, and hairstyles.

Social transitions can look very different depending on the person. Just as there are many ways we see gender expressed every day, there is considerable variety in the ways people come into transgender identities. Some may make efforts to align in dress, behavior and actions to express the gender with which they identify. This may be a gradual process, or it may move quickly.

Some individuals may choose a mash-up of styles for their gender expression or make few visible changes, and it may differ over time. The latter approach is common among nonbinary individuals—someone whose gender identity can't be described as exclusively woman or man. (Note: some nonbinary individuals do not consider themselves transgender, just nonbinary.)

There are many variations of how transgender individuals claim their identity, but the social transition focuses on how they present themselves in the world. Some transgender individuals live in this stage. Others transition in other areas as well.

Legal transition

Legal transitioning involves changing official identification of all types to align with their gender identity. Examples are changing a name and/or sex marker on documents like a driver's license, passport, Social Security record, bank accounts, etc. It can extend to birth certificates, medical records, medical insurance, or any record that typically records gender.

Changing a name on legal documents is not uncommon but changing sex markers can be complicated and varies from state to state. There are resources to help. The National Center for Transgender Equality offers self-help guides and information that can be searched by state/territory or Federal ID type.

Interestingly, as public acceptance and understanding grow, it is increasingly common to see medical portals or other online registrations offer a gender option of "other."

Medical transition

There has traditionally been a misperception that most or all transgender people desire or obtain a medical transition, which can include hormone treatment, surgery, or other actions aimed at changing the body. In fact, not all transgender people want to pursue medical transition and again, there are varying degrees. Even hormone therapy takes many forms.

Puberty blockers can be used to delay the onset of secondary sex characteristics and/or physical changes that occur during puberty, such as breast development or the enlarging of an Adam's apple. This offers an adolescent more time to learn who they are before changes occur that are harder to reverse than to delay. Once puberty blockers are stopped, puberty resumes.

Hormone therapy (HT), such as supplying estrogen, testosterone, etc., is used to alter a person's hormone levels to match their gender identity. Changes that result from hormone therapy are not as reversible, and often are not provided until an individual is older. The Mayo Clinic website has overviews of feminizing hormone therapy and masculinizing hormone therapy for more information.

Various kinds of surgery are possible as well, though surgical procedures may be less commonly used due to costs and availability. Top surgery (to reduce or enlarge breasts), voice surgery, and genital surgery are all options transgender people pursue depending on how important these issues are to them.

Summary

There is tremendous misunderstanding (and often misinformation) about what transition means. Assumptions and beliefs are often influenced by political rhetoric and legal concerns. It is important to be well-informed, because the type and degree of transition your child pursues can vary enormously.

This is a long and gradual process that may transpire over years. Let your child make their wishes known and options can be chosen in consultation with your child, your family, and your physicians and counselors.

Notes and Journaling

Telling Others

> *"What's been most difficult is the reaction of my family members. No one on my side of the family knows because our son has chosen not to tell them. He told my husband's family, but they're not supportive."*
>
> ~ Anonymous Mother from Parent Stories

Six Ways You Can Help Your Child Tell or Not Tell Others

1-Prioritize your child's needs and preferences on who and when to tell.

This story is your child's story; your child gets to decide who to tell and when to tell. They may be eager to be open, or they may be uncomfortable being discussed among family and friends. Let them take the lead or ask their permission.

2-The "big reveal" may not be necessary.

Always share in the way most helpful to your child. People may figure it out on their own and a gradual realization may be best for them. Months or years can go by without a clear statement about your child's identity while in the meantime, normal relationships are preserved.

Many people are unaware of the social stigma they express toward LGBTQ+ and transgender youth. When this becomes personal, through realizing that someone they care about is LGBTQ+, they can often find their own path to acceptance over time. Gender expressions like bright hair color, nail polish, or opposite gender dressing may simply be overlooked in someone they love.

3-If they want to be open at school, home, work, or in the family, support them all you can.

Watching your transgender loved one begin to live out their identity publicly may leave you feeling anxious. You may fear for their safety or worry about the discrimination or bullying that can occur. These realities are part of why acceptance and support at home are so important. Transgender people need a safe place—where they can talk and be heard, where they can express concerns and find encouragement, where they can be safe and find support. This is their journey, but supportive parents are a huge and valuable defense against hardships they may face. Moreover, the confidence and coping skills you help them build will serve them throughout their life.

4-They may ask you to tell someone. Help if you can.

If your child asks you to tell someone, be as helpful as you can. They may want someone to know (another parent, for example) but feel nervous about telling that person. Ask so you understand what they want you to share. If they ask, you can offer guidance to your child regarding the range of responses you anticipate.

You can accompany your child as they initiate the conversation, or you can take the lead if that is what the child wants. Be sure you understand the role they want you to play and what they want to share (or keep private).

5-They may ask you not to tell others. Respect their wishes.

The child is the one who may be the object of scrutiny, subject to questions, or a topic of family gossip. If they need privacy, let them set the pace. Coming out is their process, so the decision to tell others is theirs, not yours. This can be difficult if it means keeping a "secret" from close friends or other family members. However, the loving choice is to respect your child's needs and desires.

6-Trust your instincts—and your child's.

If you sense an acquaintance or family member may be hostile or hurtful, be mindful of this. Relatives, friends and neighbors, school chums and others all have a relationship with your child already. Again, let your child's preference lead. Try not to push them or hold them back. Be open to their reservations about certain people and honor your child's judgment.

Notes and Journaling

Relationships and Dating

> *"I was so confused and afraid when she started dating in high school. I was terrified she'd have a bad relationship or get used or settle for someone just because they were gay. Thank heavens we had older kids, so we tried to use the same rules, but it was still hard. It was years before I realized all those things happen to every kid: bad relationships, breakups, manipulative friends. I just tried to be there for her, whatever happened. But some of it was bad."*
>
> ~ Anonymous Mother from Texas

A challenging area for many parents is navigating their child's dating and romantic relationships. Every family has values and rules, and it's important to realize these do not necessarily change for a transgender child. Parents sometimes think they should handle things differently for an LGBTQ+ child, but that is seldom true. Two ideas to keep in mind:
- How would you normally handle friendships, dating, or activities?
- How have you handled them with other children in your home?

Play by the usual family rules.

As much as possible, take the transgender aspect out of the decisions you make. It can be helpful to ask yourself questions like, "Am I treating my child differently because they are transgender?" Or, "How did I (will I) handle this with my other children?" This can help ground you in the usual way your family addresses dating. This means curfews, acceptable places to go, permissions required, and responsibility can be consistent for everyone.

For non-romantic relationships, handle those similarly as well. Your child may have come out to some friends and not others. That is their choice. Allow normal school and social activities, friendships, and teams. If your child has a special interest like music, sports, academics, or animals, help them pursue it. These can help keep balance and perspective in your child's life.

Let the transgender individual set the boundaries.

Due to social or activity restrictions, some transgender youth may not come out to their group or school. They may want to avoid conflicts about sleepovers, club activity, sports teams, campouts/retreats, etc. They prefer to keep their identity private, often until a relationship or some situation arises where they feel it's important to be open. Let them set the pace. Be ready to back them when they want to be more open. By the same token, support them in coming out to people, joining activities that appeal to them, and expressing themselves as they choose, even if it feels scary to you.

Don't assume every relationship is romantic or sexual.

Like everyone else, transgender youth have friends that range from mere acquaintances to friendships to crushes. Be sure to leave room for a wide mix of relationships for your child, and don't assume every friendship is romantic. Avoid assumptions and just ask your child about friendships as you usually would. This is part of keeping communication open and helps keep their romantic interests from being an unspoken secret in the family.

Be prepared for heartache.

A common fear for parents is the loneliness their child may face in the struggle to find a romantic relationship or loving partner. While this may be a risk, their process is the same as any young person.

Finding a good partner or relationship is a challenge for everyone. Your child will be attracted to others who may or may not feel the same. They may face rejection, breakups, or heartache. There will be dates of whom you approve and others you dread. You may feel regret when a relationship ends for your child because you liked that person, or relief because you didn't care for them at all.

These are all normal events in young lives and are no different for transgender lives. As a parent, you can be an advisor, an advocate, a comfort in loss, and an encourager in need — but you can't keep these normal events from occurring. Let them find their path. Your best role is to be a safe, supportive resource as they work their way through life.

Help them find their community of people.

If possible, help your child find safe groups where they can meet or connect with other LGBTQ+ youth. Isolation leads to loneliness and despair. See our Transgender Resources list at www.strongfamilyalliance.org for possibilities and support your child in joining or participating in accepting groups. Find a trusted LGBTQ+ or transgender adult that your family can get to know as a positive role model.

Remember this is a community issue, not just a personal one. Such connections should not all be LGBTQ+ focused. For instance, the same is true of sport teams, schools, clubs, or community activities. Finding connections where your child is accepted can also provide a supportive adult community for you. If you are active in a church that is not accepting of LGBTQ+ people, it's important to consider finding a faith community that is and involving your family there.

Welcome your child's friends.

It can be very comforting to know and meet your child's friends. Providing a place for popcorn and movies or get-together activities is a great way to do so. You could host a club meeting, organize a team barbecue, or serve as a school supporter for any club or activity your child enjoys. Even something as simple as providing refreshments at a school event gives you a chance to put names to faces and get to know friends better.

An unexpected thing can sometimes occur: you become a trusted adult. If your child's friend is transgender or LGBTQ+ but not out to their own family, you may find they feel attached to you. An accepting adult may be new and hopeful to them. Be accepting but let them find their own path with their family. Do not out them, or your child, to their family if they have not chosen to do so. If a child has not come out to their family, it may not be safe for them, and coming out must always be the individual's choice.

The Importance of Names and Pronouns

One of the biggest struggles for friends and families is changing the name, and particularly the pronouns, of someone they have known so long.

Names symbolize who we are.

Names are important in our culture. Parents often name babies long before birth. Names may symbolize a dream, carry on a tradition, honor someone in the family, or show originality and alignment with a culture. For parents, changing a child's name can seem like a dismissal of all the thought and hope in the birth name. Add to that, there are years and years of habit of using a child's name.

Yet it is precisely because names are so significant that some (though not all) transgender youth change their names and ask you to use them. It may be that the chosen name symbolizes their hope of change or their view of themselves. It may be that the birth name is so associated with who they were, not who they are, that it simply doesn't fit. It may be that the birth name is painful to them, or that changing their name helps them step into their true identity. It could just be a name they love or dozens of other reasons. Whatever the reason, it is important to your child.

Some parents find it helpful to think of it as a nickname until they can get used to it. As a transition strategy that might help, but it's important to make serious and continual efforts to use their chosen name. We have all felt the tiny infraction of someone calling us by the wrong name. Socially, we usually quickly correct with a brief apology. Transgender individuals may encounter that daily, over and over, with no correction. Handle using the wrong name as you would with anyone else: a brief apology and use of the correct name.

One important thing to know is they may call the old name their "dead name". For transgender individuals who live in their identity, the use of their former name feels disrespectful, a denial of who they are, and for many, an attack. It's called "dead-naming", and is sometimes used as a form of bullying, insult, or outing an individual. Make every effort to use your child's chosen name, encourage your family to do so, and explain to them the pain dead-naming can create.

Pronouns symbolize how others see us.

Pronouns are gendered in English and many—but not all—languages. He, she, his, and hers all indicate gender. Especially when years of habit are involved, pronouns can be even harder to change than the birth name as they slip into a sentence unthinkingly. Do all you can to honor their request. Every effort you make to use the correct name or pronoun – even if you say it wrong and then correct yourself —shows support to your child.

Parents feel they are struggling to use names/pronouns; the child sees it as being supportive.

Your efforts make such an impact. Research in 2021 reinforces the positive impact your efforts can have. One important finding was that adolescents always rated their parents to be more supportive than the parents rated themselves.

While it can be a struggle to remember to use your child's new name or pronouns, understanding the importance of this action can help you as you learn.
- Their chosen name means a great deal to your child.
- Your effort to use their chosen name and pronouns is positive, even when mistakes occur.
- It gets easier with time.

Understanding they/them—plural pronouns rather than he/she, him/her, etc.

Some transgender or nonbinary individuals dislike the gendered aspects of singular pronouns like he, she, her, and him. It makes them choose an identity as either a man or a woman, when neither may feel accurate for them. This leads to the use of they/them instead, as in "I saw Josh today and they were wearing their new letter jacket."

For many people, this is a new way to think about gender, and also feels grammatically difficult. Yet it's really not uncommon when we don't know the gender of a person. For example, 'The UPS driver was here. They left the package on the porch.'

Just as with the discussion above, it's important to your child – or to other individuals you may meet – to not be mis-gendered. Do your best. It gets easier with practice. It matters and it's a constant show of acceptance to transgender people.

> *"Our finding just shows how much teens really value their parents. When we asked each group what actions they saw as showing support, parents talked about taking their teen to the gender clinic, getting them connected to resources. But what the majority of adolescents wanted most was for parents just to use their preferred name and pronoun."*
>
> ~Tandy Aye, M.D., Stanford Medicine
>
> *Associate Professor of Pediatrics*

Myths That Stigmatize Transgender People

Negative ideas about transgender individuals are often rooted in myths, stereotypes, and misinformation. Many of the LGBTQ+ myths are mistakenly equated with transgender identity because there is so much confusion between sexual orientation (who someone is attracted to) and gender identity (how someone views themselves).

Myth 1: Claiming to be transgender is:

- **a fad**
- **a choice**
- **a phase**
- **caused by peer pressure**
- **a form of rebellion.**

Reality: This is their true understanding of themselves. Transition is not an impulse or an easy change, but an effort to resolve a strong dissonance in their life and live their personal gender identity.

"Transgender people risk social stigma, discrimination, and harassment when they tell other people who they really are. Parents, friends, coworkers, classmates, and neighbors may be accepting—but they also might not be, and many transgender people fear that they will not be accepted by their loved ones and others in their life. Despite those risks, being open about one's gender identity, and living a life that feels truly authentic, can be a life-affirming and even life-saving decision." [2]

Myth 2: Children can't be transgender. It only happens at puberty.

Reality: People can realize they are transgender at any age. Much like knowing if you are right-handed or left-handed, it's hard to explain but it feels natural.

"People can realize that they're transgender at any age. Some people can trace their awareness back to their earlier memories—they just knew. Others may need more time to realize that they are transgender. Some people may spend years feeling like they don't fit in without really understanding why or may try to avoid thinking or talking about their gender out of fear, shame, or confusion. Trying to repress or change one's gender identity doesn't work; in fact, it can be very painful and damaging to one's emotional and mental health. As transgender people become more visible in the media and in community life across the country, more transgender people are able to name and understand their own experiences and may feel safer and more comfortable sharing it with others." [2]

Myth 3: All transgender people want hormone therapy and extensive surgery.

Reality: Transgender people choose to transition in many ways.

Transgender people seek transitions that make them comfortable with the way they identify. This could be clothing, grooming, mannerisms, activities, name change or many other actions that align with their view. Hormone therapy and/or surgery are sought by some but by no means all transgender individuals.

Myth 4: Transgender people hate their bodies.

Reality: Gender (body) dysphoria is not a sign of transgender identity or common to all transgender people.

"For some transgender people, the difference between the gender they are thought to be at birth and the gender they know themselves to be can lead to serious emotional distress that affects their health and everyday lives if not addressed. Gender dysphoria is a medical diagnosis for someone who experiences this distress.

Not all transgender people have gender dysphoria. On its own, being transgender is not considered a medical condition. Many transgender people do not experience serious anxiety or stress associated with the difference between their gender identity and their gender of birth, and so may not have gender dysphoria." [2]

Myth 5: The parents did something wrong.

Reality: Nothing parents did caused a child to be transgender. However, the way parents respond will have a huge impact on a child's well-being.

Self-blame is often the initial response of parents who learn that their child is transgender. This is not true. A child's gender identity is not learned from anyone, including parents. Just as a parent cannot cause a child to be heterosexual/straight/cisgender, a parent cannot cause a child to be transgender.

"At some point, nearly all children will engage in behavior associated with different genders – girls will play with trucks, boys will play with dolls, girls will hate wearing dresses and boys will insist on wearing them – and gender-nonconforming behavior does not necessarily mean that a child is transgender.

That said, sometimes these behaviors can clue us in to what a child may be feeling about their gender – with some children identifying as another gender than the one they were assigned as early as toddlerhood.

The general rule for determining whether a child is transgender or nonbinary is if the child is consistent, insistent, and persistent about their transgender identity. In other words, if your four-year-old son wants to wear a dress or says he wants to be a girl once or twice, he probably is not transgender; but if your child who was assigned male at birth repeatedly insists over the course of several months or years that she is a girl, then she is probably transgender. Children…may not have the words at a very young age to capture that feeling, but over time it may become more clear to them, and ultimately to you, that they are…a trans girl or a trans boy." [3]

Myth 6: Someone taught my child to be transgender. *OR* My child might turn other children in the family or community to be transgender.

Reality: Gender identity is not learned from peers or others.

Although children and adolescents may imitate or influence each other, gender identity is not something that is learned from peers. It is a deeply personal view of oneself rather than taking on views from someone else. Others might come out as transgender and/or LGBTQ+ to your child, not because they are "recruited," but because they recognize a common bond or shared experience of being outside social or cultural norms.

Myth 7: Transgender athletes have an advantage and should be banned from playing sports outside their gender assigned at birth.

Reality: Tens of thousands of transgender and nonbinary students have been playing sports for years without any unfair advantages or problems.

"Legislation designed to exclude transgender people, particularly women and girls, from participating in athletics has been rejected by educators, athletes, NCAA-trained facilitators, coaches, advocates for women and girls, and medical professionals. In fact, the Associated Press asked lawmakers who were seeking to pass these discriminatory bills to cite problem cases in their states and not a single lawmaker could identify a case." [4]

"The reality is that all female athletes—transgender and non-transgender—have different shapes and sizes, have different strengths and weaknesses. The research shows there's no scientific reason to exclude transgender young people. Doing so can lead to immense harm in overall well-being by interrupting an activity crucial to identity and development." [4]

> *"One doesn't have to operate with great malice to do great harm. The absence of empathy and understanding are sufficient."*
> *~ Charles M. Blow*

Myth 8: Transgender individuals could prey on women and children in public bathrooms.

Reality: Transgender people are not new, and they have been using facilities as restrooms and locker rooms consistent with their gender identity for decades without issue.

"Laws in 21 states and more than 170 cities and counties prohibit discrimination on the basis of gender identity in employment, housing, and public accommodations such as restaurants, retail establishments, and hotels. There is no evidence that these laws lead to violence or undermine safety. That is why more than 300 domestic violence and sexual assault prevention organizations support full and equal inclusion of transgender people in facilities consistent with their gender identity…Opponents of LGBTQ+ equality have admitted that their bathroom safety argument was contrived and not a real concern based on habits of actual predators." [4]

Myth 9: The Bible says God created man and woman only.

Reality: The Bible is most concerned about proper treatment of others and opposes cruelty, exploitation, and abuse among all people.

Jesus was silent on the subject of sexual orientation or gender identity. In fact, His ministry was one of welcome and acceptance to many considered outcasts or misfits, not condemnation. In addition, many Christians hold the Great Commandment in Mt. 22:36-40 as their overarching guide: "Love the Lord your God with all your heart and with all your soul and with all your mind" and "Love your neighbor as yourself."

For a more detailed discussion on scripture and transgender issues, please see "What Does the Bible Say About Transgender People."

Notes and Journaling

Meeting your LGBTQ+ child's significant other

(From Strong Family Alliance Blog)

If your child recently came out as LGBTQ+, the idea of them dating might make you pretty uncomfortable. And if the very idea makes you feel nervous and awkward, then actually meeting your child's significant other is probably not something you're prepared to do. It's not always easy, so we want to share some strategies and ideas that may help you navigate the process. Hopefully, you'll be pleasantly surprised at the outcome.

Get everyone on the same page.

First things first. In these situations, open communication is always key. Err on the side of OVER communicating. Talk to your child about their expectations and be specific. Hugs or handshakes? What does your child call their significant other? (i.e. boyfriend, girlfriend, partner, etc.) That should be the term you use in introductions.

How does your child feel about this encounter? Talk to them about how you're feeling and it's okay to say you're feeling nervous, that you're worried about saying the wrong things, etc. If you're married, how does your spouse feel about it? If you can get all these feelings and expectations out in the open before you meet, chances for success are much higher.

Don't call their significant other their "friend."

A lot of parents make the mistake of referring to their child's partner as their "friend." This happens to non-LGBTQ+ people as well and is a reflection of general parental discomfort at the idea of their "baby" being an adult. While perfectly understandable, it's even more important not to do it for your LGBTQ+ child because it sends the message that you either don't approve or don't take their relationship seriously. Use the term your child uses and practice saying it if you have to. **Remember, your child wants you to meet their partner because your approval and love is incredibly important to them.**

The fact that they're willing to have this potentially awkward experience means that they value your presence and participation in their life. Try not to take that for granted. So many LGBTQ+ people are estranged from their families and this type of situation is simply impossible. As hard as this might be for you, the fact that it can happen at all is a blessing.

Be aware of needed pronouns.

Ask your child what pronouns to use and try to use them. If you make a mistake, just quickly correct with a simple "I'm sorry" and go on. Don't make a big deal of a miss. Research shows LGBTQ+ individuals appreciate when someone tries to use the correct pronouns, even if mistakes are made. If they use certain pronouns, it can be courteous to name your own. (Hi, I'm Kate and my pronouns are she/her.")

Put yourself in their shoes.

Do you remember introducing a special someone to your family? How did it go? Were you nervous? What kinds of things did your parent or parents do/say that helped things go well (or make things super awkward)? Did those embarrassing photos from childhood make you laugh or make you want to crawl under the rug?

Let your experience guide you with your own child. LGBTQ+ people have the same kinds of hopes, desires, and challenges in their relationships as straight people, so chances are the things your parents did that made you cringe when they met your partner will also make your child uncomfortable. The same kind, welcoming words that made you feel accepted and loved will also make your child feel accepted and loved.

Your child's sexual orientation or gender identity doesn't change who they are. They're still the same child you've always loved.

Don't expect it to be perfect.

No matter how prepared you feel, odds are high that awkward moments will still happen and that's totally fine. This is a learning process. If you feel like the whole experience was a bust, you can always try again. This isn't your only chance. Make sure to check in with your child afterwards and ask how they think it went, how their partner felt, etc. Check in with yourself and your spouse.

The following questions can help everyone reflect and think about future encounters:

- o What went well?
- o What happened that felt uncomfortable or awkward?
- o What could be improved for next time?
- o Express appreciation that you had a chance to meet.

We hope these ideas will help things go more smoothly when you meet your child's significant other. Remember, someday you may meet the one that becomes a life partner, and practice now can help build awareness you'll need in the future.

REFERENCES

1. Pew Research Center. (June 13, 2013). *A survey of LGBT Americans.* http://www.pewsocialtrends.org/2013/06/13/a-survey-of-lgbt-americans/

2. National Center for Transgender Equality. (July 9, 2016). *Frequently asked questions about transgender people.* https://transequality.org/issues/resources/frequently-asked-questions-about-transgender-people

3. HRC Foundation. *Transgender children and youth: Understanding the basics.* Human Rights Campaign. https://www.hrc.org/resources/transgender-children-and-youth-understanding-the-basics.

4. HRC Foundation. *Myths and facts: Battling disinformation about transgender rights.* Human Rights Campaign. https://www.hrc.org/resources/myths-and-facts-battling-disinformation-about-transgender-rights.

Chapter 5
Coming Out as the Parent:
How Parents Can Become Allies and Advocates

Speaking Up: Independent Actions

Coming out as a parent can be gradual or sudden. As your child becomes more open, it's important that you become more open, keeping pace to provide encouragement and emotional help. Parent support begins with being an ally, a safe person to trust, but each additional step you take strengthens your child's awareness that you are with them on their journey.

> A simple, personal action we invite you to take is to share your story anonymously at Family Stories.
>
> This has several benefits:
> - **It's private** – You can share your experience anonymously.
> - **It helps you practice telling your story** — Sometimes reading our own stories gives us insight and practice telling our story that can be helpful as we eventually talk with others.
> - **It becomes a resource for others** – Parents visiting our pages can find stories from parents in similarly sized towns, geography, or family situations. You can be a help and encouragement to others.
> - **Wherever you are in your story, it can help others** -- Hearing stories from many perspectives is helpful to others finding their way.

As you take actions to be more supportive, it's important to remember this is not your story—it's your child's story. Take care to not "out" your child beyond their wishes. To help with this, we have organized suggestions in increasingly public steps. These steps help chart a path from actions that protect your child's privacy to public actions as your child becomes more public. In this guide we cover:

- Independent Actions: Coming Out as an Ally
- Going Public: Steps to Coordinate with Your Child
- Working with a Counselor: Finding Personal Support

Independent Actions: Coming Out as an Ally

There is a huge difference between acceptance/tolerance and invitation/encouragement/support…So I can be a voice that helps assure the latter becomes the norm and not the exception.
~Mother of a transgender son

Definition: Ways parents or allies can speak and act that let their community and their child know that they hold an inclusive view of LGBTQ+ people.

Why: This is showing support, whether you have an LGBTQ+ loved one or not, whether your child is publicly out or not. These actions help any LGBTQ+ person know it's safe to talk to you.

Timing: Any time

Actions you can take:

Be a Non-Participant

- Refuse to participate in subtle or overt LGBTQ+ disparagement.
    - Do not use negative language, tease, or make disrespectful jokes.
    - Walk away from disparaging conversations.

Express an Inclusive Attitude

- Make proactive efforts to discuss LGBTQ+ people and ideas.
    - Avoid silence. Silence makes LGBTQ+ topics seem taboo.
- Find opportunities to talk about LGBTQ+ people or issues in positive ways.

    - Talk about LGBTQ+ individuals you know and what you admire about them (co-workers, friends, relatives, etc.).
    - Discuss news stories or current events around LGBTQ+ issues (same-sex marriage, bathroom bills, discrimination, health issues, news, etc.).
    - Comment on celebrities, politicians, or advocates who are or who support LGBTQ+ and why that matters.

Outreach

- Establish relationships with LGBTQ+ people in your community.
    - Encourage LGBTQ+ youth that you encounter through sports, friendships, school, etc. Be friendly and normal to these youth as you would to any others.
    - Extend invitations to shared activities such as inviting an LGBTQ+ neighbor to dinner or a movie or asking someone to join a league or group activity (sports, music, gardening, cooking, etc.).

Take a Stand

- Confront others' negative word/actions.
    - Object to derogatory comments or jokes ("That's a hurtful comment", "That's not funny").
    - Correct your child (or siblings, or relatives) for negative comments.
    - Criticize negative examples of such behavior in movies, TV, news stories, etc.

- Be a public advocate.
    - Donate to organizations that promote LGBTQ+ rights.
    - Participate in demonstrations in your area.
    - Vote for inclusive office holders.
    - Encourage your church, temple, or mosque to support LGBTQ+ members.

Come Out Anonymously

- Learn all you can.

    o Get factual information, resources and suggestions from supportive websites such as strongfamilyalliance.org or pflag.org/transgender.
    o Read about others' stories of being a parent of an LGBTQ+ person (e.g., "Family Stories" at strongfamilyalliance.org).
    o For an informative and encouraging article about transgender youth and their families, visit "How Parents Can Best Support a Transgender Child: Research Study" (YouTube: Where Parents Talk TV).

- Share your own story in a private, confidential way.

    o Add your story anonymously online at "Family Stories" on our website.
    o Find confidential, private support.
    o Work with an affirming knowledgeable therapist.
    o Talk with supportive, accepting clergy.
    o Join a support group such as PFLAG.

Notes and Journaling

Going Public: Steps to Coordinate with Your Child

Remember:

- It's not your story to tell—you will not feel the scrutiny, your child will.
- Keep pace with your child—their comfort level is most important.
- Get permission—ask if you can talk to a particular person (even your sibling or best friend).
- Judge your audience—they may break confidence or gossip.

Definition: The timing of telling friends, family, or anyone that your child identifies as transgender and/or LGBTQ+ is important. This is complex and must be based on your child's decisions of who knows and when.

Why: Keeping pace with your child is a way to support your child, find support yourself, and become an advocate.

Timing: Depends on your child's comfort level. Becoming completely open could happen quickly, or it may take years, or it may never occur. You must take cues from your child about whom to tell and when.

Protecting Privacy: Child Is Only Out to You

- Caution: Do not "out" your child.
    - However emotional you are, respect your child's privacy. Take time to find your balance and gather helpful information.
- Be an ally.
    - See the independent actions above and pursue all you can.

- Educate yourself.
    - This is support for you as well and there are many options (e.g., PFLAG, TransFamilies.org, strongfamilyalliance.org/resources).
- Find a confidential and supportive space.
    - Join a support group such as PFLAG or one of the many affirming faith-based resources.
    - Online groups can be especially helpful, such as those from the TransFamilies.org website which hosts events in both English and Spanish.
    - Work with an affirming therapist.
    - Talk with accepting clergy.
- Tell your story anonymously
    - Post your anonymous story on our website at strongfamilyalliance.org/Family Stories.

Assisting and Asking Permission: Child Told a Trusted Few

- Keep pace.
    - Don't ask your child to stretch and don't hold them back.
- If asked, be willing to help tell others.
    - Help your child tell someone else if your child wants your help. You may be part of the conversation, or you may be sent as a messenger.
- Ask permission if you want to tell someone.
    - For someone your child knows well, such as a relative or close friend, it's essential your child agrees. It's their relationship too.
- Ask how you can help.
    - Sometimes they want help and other times not. It's important to ask, so they stay in control.
- Keep the conversation flowing.
    - Ask normal questions about life, school, work, and friends. Don't make everything about being LGBTQ+.
- Keep your worries to yourself.
    - Find a trusted resource to talk with but don't lay your fears on your child.

Acknowledging and Educating Others: Child Is Out to Some Family or Friends

- Be a welcoming home.
    - Invite their friends to your home. Make an effort to know ALL their friends, but particularly those close to your child.
- Find your comfort zone.
    - Practice talking about this change until you have the words comfortably down.
- Ask your child how to handle questions.
    - Find out how they answer and parallel them.
- Be a buffer if needed.
    - Keep your balance if someone else such as a relative is emotional or critical. Don't let them grill your child.
- Discuss possible gossip.
    - Help your child be realistic that others may talk. Take your cue from your child.
- Get your statements and answers down pat.
    - Find positive, affirming ways to answer if someone asks or implies something. You are an ally—act like it.

Creating Normalcy and Ease: Child Is Progressively Open

- Grow with your child.
    - Be more open as your child is more open. Talk easily about this and many other topics around school, activities, sports, etc.
- Be ready for dating and relationships.
    - Try to apply consistent guidelines about dating. Curfews, activities, and boundaries can still be appropriate.
    - There may be open affection. Try to think "if they were a co-ed couple would this bother me?"
- Make your home a destination.
    - You can become a friend to others whose families may be rejecting or on the same journey.

Speaking Up: Both You and Your Child Are Out

- Take a public stand.
    - Join one of the many support and advocacy groups you can find listed on our website.
- Advocate
    - Actively advocate for LGBTQ+ rights. Be a public voice when possible.
- Help other families and youth.
    - Support or help your school start a GSA Club.
    - Recommend GLSEN resources to teachers and school counselors.
    - Be available to parents with a child coming out as a support. Help them find resources and information.

Notes and Journaling

Working with a Counselor: Finding Personal Support

People are often hesitant to see a counselor, or therapist, particularly if this is the first time to reach out. Below are some common questions and answers about counseling.

Definition: Share thoughts, feelings, questions, and concerns about being the parent of an LGBTQ+ child either anonymously (e.g., online) or with a therapist who is bound by confidentiality.

Why: It can be helpful to discuss experiences with others to who may offer support, information, and insight.

Timing: Any time.

Why therapy?

Therapy can help when you've tried everything and still notice that stress, change, difficulties, or feelings…
…are unmanageable
…are not getting better with time
…are getting in the way of your roles and duties in life (e.g., at work, as a parent, or with everyday activities)

In other words, therapy is a way to find relief when things are beyond your ability to cope, not resolving despite time and effort, and creating impairment in your life.

Also, therapy is appropriate in times of growth, exploration, confusion, and adjustment to new ideas and identities, even when things are good!

Parents of kids who have come out as LGBTQ+ may find that they move through each of these experiences and need a place to bring all the pieces together.

How can it help?

Therapy can be many things and is tailored to what you want. It can be a place to get unstuck, find new understanding of yourself and others, process painful memories or feelings, learn new skills and tools, and get inspired to make exciting changes in yourself or your relationships. Specifically for parents of kids who identify as LGBTQ+, therapy is a private place to air reactions of fear, doubt, or confusion and ask questions.

Isn't it just talking with someone?

Even the good listeners in your life are not able to listen with nonjudgment, focusing only on your best interests. Most friends and family members struggle to hear difficult feelings such as anger, sadness, or shame without trying to solve problems or minimize feelings. Therapists join with your struggle and help in a way that is effective, respectful, and confidential.

What's the difference between counseling and therapy?

These words are essentially interchangeable.

How do I find a therapist?

1. Get several names of local therapists to research. Some ways to do this:
    - Ask your doctor for recommendations.
    - If you have a health insurance plan, call the customer service number on your card and ask for help finding a list of "in-network mental health providers."
    - Search the Psychology Today Therapist Finder for your zip code, your concern, or your insurance plan. (Not all therapists choose to be listed here, but many do.)
    - Use online resources such as betterhelp.com or where you can set criteria and preview therapists.
    - Since the events around COVID, even local therapists may offer online sessions

2. Find out more about the therapists. Some questions to ask or research:
   - Are they accepting new clients?
   - Are they inclusive and experienced with LGBTQ+ clients and concerns?
   - What are the fees? Do they accept insurance?
   - Do they provide individual therapy? Couples? Family? Child therapy?

(Note: Letters such as PhD, LPC, LMFT, and LCSW represent the type of training and licensure the therapist obtained, but these letters will not determine who feels like a good match or who will work most effectively with you.)

Are there two or three questions I could ask to make sure they are inclusive and competent to work with concerns related to my LGBTQ+ child and our family?

Your goal is to find a counselor who is knowledgeable and affirming, which is very different from friendly and accepting. You could ask if a therapist specializes or has experience working with LGBTQ+ concerns. Be wary of any therapist who claims to "fix" or "cure" being gay or transgender, as this will not be a good fit. Other good indicators are whether paperwork or other written material on their website reflect sexual and gender diversity/ For example, the website mentions "transgender "or "LGBTQ" in a description of services on their website, has inclusive choices for gender on intake paperwork, provides links to inclusive resources, etc.

Why would I go just for me?

You cannot change others' reactions, choices, or experiences, but you can work to understand and even change your own. You are worthy of good self-care, and therapy is part of that. If it is difficult to justify something only for yourself, remind yourself that as you benefit, most likely your loved ones will benefit indirectly as well. Although self-care is reason enough, improving mental wellness in order to improve parenting may motivate some parents to seek therapy.

Should I go even if my spouse won't?

Therapy is a personal and individual decision. You can benefit even if your partner does not attend.

Should I consider counseling for my child?

Yes. If you think that your child is struggling, offering or encouraging individual therapy could be a good idea. Family therapy can also be a way to strengthen relationships and communication with your child. Offer, invite, and encourage therapy if you feel it is the right step; however, forcing therapy on an adolescent who is not willing or ready can cause strain and stress.

How do I find the right therapist and make sure they'll work well with my child?

The process is the same as described previously, with one addition: listen to your child regarding whether they feel comfortable with the therapist. Some kids need a few sessions to feel comfortable and establish rapport with the therapist. Other kids and teens begin to balk at therapy after several sessions, when topics may get more difficult or personal. These issues are normal and something to bring up with the therapist, so they can monitor rapport and engagement. However, regardless of whether the child enjoys the process of therapy, a relationship with the therapist in which they feel respected, understood, and heard by the therapist is of the utmost importance. Consider giving your child the ability to look at a few websites and decide who they will see. This reinforces their sense of independence and choice.

Should we try family therapy?

Yes, if you notice that the way your family handles problems, conflicts, and changes is not working well. A family therapist does not focus on the problems of one person, but rather focuses on the way family members interact as a group.

When would I use group therapy or individual therapy?

Both can provide a sense of relief that you are not alone. Group therapy can be a powerful way to understand yourself through relationships with and the support of others. It has many of the same benefits as individual therapy and is often less expensive. In some cases, individual therapy may be needed before group therapy if working toward feeling stable or functioning in daily life activities are primary goals.

We don't have insurance coverage. Where can we get help?

Community mental health agencies often have a "sliding scale" fee structure that allows for paying what is affordable to you, based on your income. Support groups can also be a lower cost option.

How long does counseling go on?

This depends on you, the therapist, and the goals you set together. Terminating therapy is best approached as a joint decision between client and therapist, but clients can decide to discontinue therapy at any time. However, a question to ask a therapist in the first session or two is how long they anticipate the work will last. Some therapists work within a short-term therapy model, others allow for ongoing, start-and-stop work, and others form treatment plans that estimate the number of sessions needed.

How much will it cost?

If you are not using health insurance, "private pay" rates for 50–60-minute sessions can range widely, anywhere from $80 to $175 or higher, in some cases. Group therapy sessions usually range from $20 to $50 per meeting.

Can I choose what I ask for help on?

Yes! You are in charge of what concerns and goals you bring to therapy. A therapist may recommend exploring other things, but your primary concerns should drive therapy goals.

I live in a small town. Is there any way I can get help online or remotely?

Telehealth or telemedicine, e-therapy, or online therapy as it is sometimes called, has become increasingly common. Including search terms such as "online therapy" or "teletherapy" will reveal a list of therapy providers that provide this service.

I'm a Christian. Can I find a Christian counselor?

Yes. Some counselors indicate online or in other materials that they focus in that area. This designation usually means the counselor is a Christian—not that they are qualified to give theological answers.

It's important to make sure they are able to help you support your LGBTQ+ child and are not condemning. A direct question before making an appointment might be "Are they affirming/accepting/supportive of LGBTQ+ individuals?"

If I'm a Christian, can I see a non-Christian counselor?

Of course. Counselors help clients address emotional or mental needs of many types: concerns, decisions, emotional struggles, relationship problems, etc. For parents of an LGBTQ+ child, there are many concerns separate from religious questions where a counselor can assist. If your faith is not accepting of LGBTQ+ individuals, a non-religious counselor may be the best option and provide additional insights. They may also be more able to address concerns around your child's safety, friends, activities, and social interests.

When would I see a pastor versus a counselor?

This is partly a personal preference. If you are close to a pastor and trust them to be supportive of your LGBTQ+ child, they may be a good resource. (Pastors who are not supportive would hopefully point you to other alternatives.) Often people prefer to see a counselor rather than a pastor for more privacy. It can be hard to interact with a pastor socially or in services when you are in active counseling with them. Sometimes people find that seeing both is a better answer than either/or. That allows them to work on theology and faith issues with the pastor and personal struggles with the counselor.

If I can't find or afford a therapist, what can I do? (Journaling? Reading? etc.?)

Many therapists offer sliding scale rates, and some agencies offer therapy for free or at a reduced cost. Additionally, local or online support groups can be a place to interact with others who have similar experiences. Journaling and reading self-help books or online resources can be helpful in the meantime. You can find additional books in our resources list on our website.

Notes and Journaling

Chapter 6
Moving Forward

> *"I'm 5 years into parenting an LGBTQ+ child, but I continue to learn. The issues change over time (safety, bullying, health, dating, college, roommates, partners, etc.) but I find I get better at it. What was hard at first has become so much easier. And finding good resources is such a gift."*
> ~Father of a gay son

Tough Questions

Below are some hard questions parents often ask and answers that can be helpful. There are many other sources for frequently asked questions but here we focus on questions often not answered elsewhere.

Why is suicide emphasized so much as a risk?

Because suicide is the highest risk of death for transgender and LGBTQ+ individuals.

Because most teen suicides are impulsive with little or no planning and 70% occur in the victim's homes.[3]

As a cause of death, suicide is:

- 12th leading cause of death in the US[1]
- 3rd leading cause of death among US teens[2]
- 1st cause of death among gay and lesbian youth[3]
- The suicide attempts among transgender persons ranges from 32% to 50% across the countries.[4]

SPEAK also provides warning signs to look for:[3]

- Giving away prized possessions
- Feelings of worthlessness or guilt
- Change in eating habits and sleep patterns
- Extreme personality changes
- Aggressive, destructive, or defiant behavior
- Neglect of personal appearance or hygiene
- Increase in alcohol or drug consumption
- Talking, writing, or drawing about their own death
- Withdrawing from family or friends

Who are we now? As parents? As a family?

Although it may feel as if everything has changed, in most ways you are the same family you have been. The child who comes out to you is the same person you loved moments before. Daily decisions and activities may change gradually but try to take time, keep normal routines as much as possible, allow things to settle into new patterns gradually, and focus on communication and affection.

Let us offer some reassurance. On our parent stories page, you can search on transgender stories. One of the last questions we ask is: Knowing what you know today, would you want your child to "stay in the closet"? Why?

In story after story the answer is "No". The reasons may vary, but the general answers are because their child is happier and their family stronger for having weathered this change together. We hope you find this true as well.

What about my dreams and expectations?

You've probably imagined possible futures for your child that seem out of reach now. The death of dreams and shattered expectations may be hard to bear but try to focus on the bigger picture. Parents hope for many things for a child: good health, a happy life, close friends, a good education, a job, a loving relationship, a way to serve in the world, and many more.

All of these can still be dreams, though the details of how they occur may differ. Dream big for your child—maybe dream bigger than ever before. They need your hopeful view and encouragement.

Will my child have a lonely, miserable life?

You might be worrying that this means no marriage partnership, no children, or no happiness. Despite your own fears, it's important to help your child dream a positive future. For LGBTQ+ individuals, hopelessness can breed self-destructive behaviors and despair can breed suicidal thoughts.

To help counteract this risk, one of the most important things a parent can do is hold a hopeful view of the future and share that with their child. And the truth is, many, many LGBTQ+ people lead productive, connected lives with loving partners and families.

Sometimes a minor shift in your own dream can help and basic dreams still hold:
- The dream of a great spouse for your child is at heart the hope for a good partner, one who loves and supports your child.
- Loneliness is greatly counterbalanced by strong family connections—which you can help sustain.

Check out *It Gets Better*, either the book or website. Both are full of encouraging stories that can help you build a positive vision of the future. Your child can also find encouragement there as well.

I want to tell my closest friend/relative. Should I?

It may feel strange not telling a close friend. You may really need to talk with someone about what you are feeling. Your needs are important, but you have to carefully choose where you find support and find a safe place to talk. Very few people come out to their parent and the world in the same day. It's a gradual process over time, and you have to be patient and let that unfold.

You want the family to allow the child to remain in control of the story and how it spreads. Telling too many people is like spilling glitter – you can't get it all back in the bottle.

Consider these points:

- When you tell someone, you are "outing" your child. Consider whether your child will be exposed to comments, opinions, scrutiny, gossip.

- If it's a relative or someone the child knows well, your child has a relationship with them as well. It's even more important for your child to be comfortable with them knowing.

- You may wonder if people notice differences, but many may not know or notice changes in your family. As your transgender child's transition progresses -- as appearance and names/pronouns change --you are able to be more open because your child is more open. Keep pace.

Finally, remember this is not your story to tell. It's your child's story. It is imperative to let the child decide when they are ready to come out and to whom. You must be your child's protector by doing what your child needs in terms of openness or privacy. Your story is your own experience, but your role as a parent involves supporting your child in the degree of openness comfortable for them.

Will I have grandchildren?

Many parents long for grandchildren and you may think having a transgender or LGBTQ+ child means you won't have grandchildren. This will be your child's choice, just as it would be in any relationship. They may conceive, adopt, foster, or choose not to parent. Don't assume the outcome. Let time play out the situation, just as it would in any partner relationship.

How do I decide when to tell people?

It differs depending on the situation. But as a rule, you let your child decide who knows what and when. Don't "out" them to someone unless your child says that it is OK with them.

What is the "second closet?

The term "in the closet" refers to the choice that transgender and LGBTQ+ individuals make to keep their identity to themselves. Family members are said to be in the "second closet" when they are keeping the child's identity private from others in the family or community. The second closet can be either a positive or a negative situation and it's vital that those trusted by the child understand the difference.

It is positive if the child is deciding who knows and when, and those trusted are abiding by the child's desire for privacy or openness. You are supporting their preference and allowing them to control their experience.

It is negative if the child is ready to be more open and the family resists. This makes the child the "family secret." For the child, this can feel like rejection, rebuff the trust the child showed through their honesty, and instill a sense that their family is ashamed.

It can be difficult to find the right step in each situation but asking your child and keeping pace with their wishes are key.

How do I deal with my child dating someone whose parents don't know their child is transgender or LGBTQ+?

As a rule, each child's decision to come out must be their own. If the other young person is not out to their family, they may not be ready, or it may not be safe for them at home. You are not obligated to tell others that your child is transgender or LGBTQ+, or that their child is. You can encourage the child to tell their parents when they are ready and offer to help in any way you can with that step, but to tell the parents without the child's permission could damage multiple relationships.

If you encounter criticism from the other parent later (why didn't you tell me?), you may be faced with a tough conversation. Be as honest as you can about your reasoning and up front about any difficulty you may have felt around the choice to remain silent. It may be helpful to share that although in many cases your policy is to inform other parents when things arise with their child, sharing about a child's identity before they are ready can be hurtful to the child.

Even after explaining that protecting the child's privacy is ultimately a choice to protect the child, the other parent may not understand. The choice to prioritize a child's wishes, privacy, and potentially their safety over harmony with that child's parent is not an easy position to take, but ultimately this is what we recommend.

Do I have to tell my church or house of worship?

No, but telling depends on the church. There are affirming faith communities of all religions. (See Faith-Based Organizations at www.strongfamilyalliance.org.) However, if your family is closely connected to a faith community, rejection by that community can be damaging, particularly if the child feels judged.

If you anticipate judgmental reactions, it may no longer be a good place for your family. Consider finding a more accepting faith community. If you decide to stay and your child is wounded by the church, the risk is that your child may eventually come to question or even reject his or her faith entirely.

Why did my child tell me?

You may almost wish you didn't know. The good news is children decide to tell their parents for good reasons. They may long to remove hidden barriers and to be accepted for who they are. Many wish to be honest with their family and may feel they have lived a lie with the people they cherish most. Their openness is an act of courage and shows deep trust in you. Try to honor them for honoring you with the truth.

Should I encourage my child to hide their transgender identity to keep them safe?

Coming out is a very personal decision, but recent research shows it is better for them to come out when they are ready rather than hide when they are wanting to be more open. A 2015 study, entitled Coming Out at School and Well-being in Young Adulthood,[5] found hiding their identity did not keep them safe and had other negative consequences. Key findings were:

- LGBTQ+ students experienced school victimization regardless of whether they attempted to conceal their identity or openly disclosed their LGBT identity. Thus, hiding was not successful, on average, in protecting LGBTQ+ students from school victimization and bullying.

- LGBTQ+ young adults who tried to hide their sexual orientation and gender identity at school reported more victimization and, ultimately, higher levels of depression than LGBTQ+ students who came out or were open about their LGBTQ+ identity at school. Feeling that they had to hide their sexual orientation and gender identity was associated with depression among LGBTQ+ young adults.
- Being out about one's LGBTQ+ identity at school has strong associations with self-esteem and life satisfaction and with low levels of depression in young adulthood.

Your child's decision is of primary importance. Your efforts to support them is a close second.

Why do other teens shame or shun my child?

This can be complex. Unfortunately, it can be a frequent experience in schools. There may be many reasons, but some common ones are:

- **Peer pressure**—Teens long for a sense of belonging, which may come with feeling "the same as" their friends. They may avoid someone they learn is LGBTQ+ simply because they are different.

- **Fear of association**—"They'll think I'm gay/trans/etc. too." Because of the anti-LGBTQ+ messages in our society, peers may worry others will make assumptions about them too.

- **Condemnation by their families or church**—They may be reflecting what they have heard or been taught. Kids often voice the values and beliefs of their parents, and when parents make statements against the gay community, their kids may too.

- **Projection**—Sometimes people who are LGBTQ+ (and are uncomfortable with this) deny their own feelings and accuse others of having those very feelings. It can be a way of avoiding suspicion and diverting attention to others.

- **Deflection**—Gossiping about someone who is LBGTQ+ to test other people's reactions. This tactic allows kids to preview what might happen if they were to come out.

- **Otherness**—Emphasizing the "difference" factor. Unfortunately, it is human nature to confirm an idea of ourselves as "good" or "right" by calling out someone else as "bad" or "wrong." Adolescents especially are looking for belonging and/or fitting in.

- **Prurience**—Focus on sexual activity rather than the person. Adolescent, who are often preoccupied with sex, may be especially prone to ignore the whole person and focus solely on their sexuality.

Please see www.glsen.org for information on bullying and school programs. For additional or more general questions visit:

www.pflag.org
www.advocatesforyouth.org
www.belongto.org
www.aids.nlm.nih.gov

Issues of Faith

For many people who are a part of a religion or faith, there may be a conflict between some beliefs...
- "Homosexuality is a sin"
- Opposition to gay marriage
- LGBTQ+ people should not be ordained or work in a church
- Two genders, "male" and "female," were created by God

AND your belief that...
- "My child is a good person"
- "My child is a beloved child of God"
- My faith's writings emphasize love and service above all
- My child identifies and expresses themselves as God created them

We have suggestions that can help.

Hit the pause button
You don't have to decide right now how to reconcile every question. Most religions reject the notion that children are a parent's property and have strong teachings on the importance of family cohesion. Focus on keeping the family intact and allow time to work through faith struggles.

Lead with love
This is the same child you have loved and cherished for years. Keep leading with love as it may help you carve out space to resolve other issues over time. Most religions emphasize parent roles and almost universally maintain that the most important parental obligation is the obligation to love one's children.

Keep being the best parent you possibly can
Prioritize staying close to your child to maintain the safety, support, and interaction so essential as they grow to adulthood. They still need parenting, encouragement, love and safety at home.

Resist being swayed by judgment
If you feel judgment from others about your child, or you struggle with your own judgment about what it means to be LGBTQ+, put your relationship with your child first. Maintain communication and affection that is so important for a family relationship.

Represent your faith
Remember your daily example is a living demonstration of your faith for your child. Focusing on the overarching beliefs of their faith such as love, kindness, healing, and devotion to God helps many who struggle with individual negative scriptures.

Find support
You may be wondering how or whether to talk about this with others who share your religion. Find a supportive person to help you decide if it is safe for you and your child to discuss it. If you have concerns about your own church, consider reading some of the books in our Resources list at www.strongfamilyalliance.org or reaching out to another church.

Protect privacy
Depending on your relationship with your church, its leaders, or the community you may feel like you are keeping a secret. This may be necessary to protect your child from unwanted scrutiny and judgment.

Seek positive resources in your denomination
Almost every denomination or religion has supportive groups for LGBTQ+ people and often provides new ways to think about these changes in the family. If you have doubts or your church is condemning, please visit our "Faith Based Organizations" page at www.strongfamilyalliance.org to find references for your denomination.

Use prayer
Many people learn over time that their relationship with God can take many forms. Parents of transgender or LGBTQ+ children often pray their way through parenting. Finding a one-on-one faith interaction can guide their daily actions better than written rules in their faith.

Help your child keep their faith
Perhaps the most important point is that youth raised in a faith often have deep spiritual longings for faith connections. Staying in a condemning church may drive your child away from faith entirely. Finding a spiritual home that accepts the entire family may be the single greatest gift of faith, witness, and guidance you can provide.

Notes and Journaling

Valuable Resources

Most parents learn as they go along, and each family's path is unique. Good resources are available and it's helpful to know how to find them. From research reports to health information to support groups we encourage you to use these widely available tools to answer questions.

Below are some key ones that can provide safe and reputable resources. Links for these are at www.strongfamilyalliance.org.

Support & Advocacy

Here you'll find a listing of key organizations providing education and information by and for transgender and LGBTQ+ people, their families, and their allies. There are sections for:
- Key support and advocacy groups
- Research sources
- Education and school support and materials
- Tips for college bound students
- Civil rights and laws
- Major religions

Faith-Based Organizations

In almost every faith group, there are resources for support. Our list includes:
- Christian (22 Denominations)
- Non-denominational
- Buddhist
- Hindu
- Islam
- Judaism
- Ecumenical

Books

Titles include parenting, the coming out experience, LGBT resources, transgender resources, as well as Christian and Jewish writers.

Resources

Find recent blogs, video, news and articles and a parent forum where you can post issues or questions for other parents to answer.

Finding Medical Resources

It is vitally important to get help and get accurate information. Your child is making decisions about how they want to present to the world, but it is sometimes hard to know when to help and when to act with caution. Accurate information for families is constantly expanding and can be invaluable for you and your transgender child.

Work With a Supportive Physician. Please talk with your pediatrician about the concerns you have. Medical advice may resolve many questions. However, it's essential your physician is accepting of LGBTQ+ patients and there are resources to help locate providers. Here are some national resources to assist:

- The Human Rights Campaign publishes a listing of healthcare facilities throughout the United States that promote equitable and inclusive care for LGBTQ+ and their families. (Search for Healthcare Equality Index for the most recent report.)
- The "Transgender Care Listing" at transcaresite.org allows you to use qualifiers for practice type and location to find a provider.
- The GLMA is the world's largest and oldest association of lesbian, gay, bisexual, transgender and queer (LGBTQ) healthcare professionals. Medical professionals must self-list.

Helpful Resources for Other Information

Kids In The House is an extensive website for parenting information on a broad range of topics. Search under transgender to find dozens of videos from parents and experts, a wealth of articles and a forum.

The National Center for Transgender Equality's "About Transgender People" has a primer of basic transgender information and links to other resources.

The Mayo Clinic offers a helpful "Transgender Facts" page on their website.

GLAAD provides "Tips for Allies of Transgender People" with frequent questions, tips for allies, and a list of links to more resources.

The PFLAG transgender resource page offers a reading list as well as information on a number of legal, social and political issues affecting transgender persons.

A final note:

We hear repeatedly from parents that working through the changes of a child coming out can be hard but results in deeper, closer relationships. With our very best wishes, we hope that is true for your family as well.

How to Have a More Meaningful Holiday
by Janet Gattis Duke
(From Strong Family Alliance Blog)

Each holiday dinner, we encourage our gay child to bring along any LGBTQ+ friends that might not have a place to go. For nearly twenty years there have always been guests. Young people alone at Thanksgiving or Christmas or July 4. Once we had five visitors, always it's one or two. Some come once, a few come several times.

There is food, of course, but we also have games and puzzles and serial football to watch. A few I have met before, but most are strangers to me. It surprised me to realize some were near strangers to my daughter as well—a friend of a friend—but they were alone, so she invited. Some are pierced and tattooed. Some are in polos and slacks. Some reserved, others outgoing, but most relax as the day passes.

We don't ask why they are separated from their family, why they are alone. Rather we have the interesting conversations that can happen with someone you just meet. We talk about movies, current events, school, hobbies. I remember laughing conversations about learning to drive, their best Halloween costume, beloved pets, and their worst camping experiences.

Often life challenges come up. They talk about car break downs, struggles to finish college while working, apartment robberies, or credit card nightmares. As our visitors have gotten older conversations include job hunting, worries about conflicts with bosses or co-workers, money management, and dreams of owning a house. We are sometimes asked for advice. My husband might help diagnose a car problem. We might talk about budgeting or what percent of income should go to housing.

I enjoy these days and the many young men and women I've met. But I also hurt for them and their families. Those parents who are missing in action. The siblings who aren't close because a gay child has been cast out. They should be the ones laughing at the humorous stories, learning small details about the everyday lives of their child. The parents should be hearing about struggles in work or school, helping with problems, comforting if the child has been robbed or attacked. But they are missing in action.

I am struck each time at the loss on both sides, the break in family support and family connection. It is so harmful to everyone.

I remember one woman turning to me as I walked her to the door after a fun, sunny afternoon of food and companionship. She turned and spoke in a slightly choked voice, saying thank you, then, "I haven't been in a family home since my parents kicked me out when I was 14. It was really good to be here."
She was 24. Ten years. A decade.

What her parents have missed. They don't know this poised, eloquent, caring woman who volunteers with the animal shelter and works for an architect. They don't know her hopes and dreams, her struggles and successes. They don't know their child's life. Because they are missing in her life.

This holiday season bring your LGBTQ+ loved ones home, bring their friends as well, start building new memories around family and holidays. It's never too soon—and it's never too late—to remember that family is forever.

REFERENCES

1. American Foundation for Suicide Prevention. *Suicide Statistics.* https://afsp.org/suicide-statistics/ Accessed on May 25, 2022.

2. Minino, A. M. (May 2010). *Mortality among teenagers aged 12-19 years: United States, 1999-2006.* Hyattsville, MD: National Center for Health Statistics, Data Brief No. 37. Centers for Disease Control and Prevention. https://www.cdc.gov/nchs/products/databriefs/db37.htm

3. SPEAK: Suicide Prevention Awareness Education for Kids. *Suicide facts.* http://www.speakforthem.org/facts.html.

4. Virupaksha, H. G., Muralidhar, D., & Ramakrishna, J. (2016). Suicide and suicidal behavior among transgender persons. *Indian Journal of Psychological Medicine, 38(6),* 505–509. https://doi.org/10.4103/0253-7176.194908

5. Family Acceptance Project. (March 25, 2015). *Coming out at school and well-being in young adulthood.* https://familyproject.sfsu.edu/news-announce/coming-out-school-and-well-being-young-adulthood.

About the Authors

Janet Gattis Duke, Founder Strong Family Alliance

Janet's lesbian daughter came out over two decades ago. Strong Family Alliance is her effort to provide others the information, guidance and resources she longed for to keep her child safe and her family strong. She also serves on the board of the Reconciling Ministries Network working for full inclusion of LGBTQ+ in all aspects of the United Methodist Church, and on the board of the Parents Reconciling Network, supporting parents of LGBTQ+ children.

Janet spent 35 years with IBM where her work with international teams gave her a deep appreciation of racial, cultural, and social diversity. Retiring from IBM, she worked 10 years for the non-profit Service Dogs Inc. Retiring from that (she has a problem retiring), she now focuses on LGBTQ+ family issues and enjoys hiking, time in the mountains, and working to certify her Labrador as a therapy dog.

Shailagh Clarke, Ph.D.

Shailagh Clarke, Ph.D. is the first board member of Strong Family Alliance. As a licensed psychologist in private practice, Shailagh has seen first-hand the struggle families experience when a child comes out. Her vision is that the Strong Family web site will be a resource that will help preserve these families.

She obtained her master's degree and Ph.D. from the University of North Texas and bachelor's degree in Plan II and Psychology from the University of Texas at Austin.

Shailagh lives in Lakeway, Texas with her partner and three children. After spending most of her life avoiding sports, she now enjoys playing tennis regularly.

Jennifer Gamewell, M.Ed, LPC, CCST, CPDPE

Jennifer (pronouns she/her/hers) obtained her bachelor's degree from The University of Texas, Austin and spent twenty years as a school counselor, primarily working within the middle school environment. During her time as a school counselor, she attended Texas A&M University earning a Master's Degree in Educational Psychology, which enabled her to start her own private practice in 2017, Gamewell Innovative Counseling, LLC.

Jennifer is highly experienced in assisting families, young adults, adolescents, and children with developmental, behavioral, social, and emotional issues. She provides gender affirming therapy for individuals who may be transgender, nonbinary, or at any point along the gender spectrum. Her professional specialization involves working with individuals who are questioning, exploring, accepting, clarifying, or adapting to their identity.

Printed in Great Britain
by Amazon